Strength and Conditioning

Special Issue Editor

Lee E. Brown

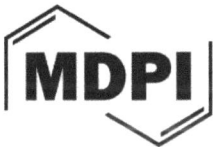

Special Issue Editor
Lee E. Brown
Center for Sport Performance
California State University
USA

Editorial Office
MDPI AG
St. Alban-Anlage 66
Basel, Switzerland

This edition is a reprint of the Special Issue published online in the open access journal *Sports* (ISSN 2075-4663) from 2015–2016 (available at: http://www.mdpi.com/journal/sports/special_issues/strength-conditioning).

For citation purposes, cite each article independently as indicated on the article page online and as indicated below:

Author 1; Author 2; Author 3 etc. Article title. *Journalname*. **Year**. Article number/page range.

ISBN 978-3-03842-346-1 (Pbk)
ISBN 978-3-03842-347-8 (PDF)

Table of Contents

About the Guest Editor...v

Preface to "Strength and Conditioning"...vii

Jason B. White, Trevor P. Dorian and Margaret T. Jones
Lateral Squats Significantly Decrease Sprint Time in Collegiate Baseball Athletes
Reprinted from: *Sports* **2016**, 4(1), 19; doi: 10.3390/sports4010019
http://www.mdpi.com/2075-4663/4/1/19 1

Pablo B. Costa, Trent J. Herda, Ashley A. Herda and Joel T. Cramer
Effects of Short-Term Dynamic Constant External Resistance Training and Subsequent Detraining
on Strength of the Trained and Untrained Limbs: A Randomized Trial
Reprinted from: *Sports* **2016**, 4(1), 7; doi: 10.3390/sports4010007
http://www.mdpi.com/2075-4663/4/1/7 10

Taylor S. Thurston, Jared W. Coburn, Lee E. Brown, Albert Bartolini, Tori L. Beaudette,
Patrick Karg, Kathryn A. McLeland, Jose A. Arevalo, Daniel A. Judelsonand Andrew J. Galpin
Effects of Respiratory Muscle Warm-up on High-Intensity Exercise Performance
Reprinted from: *Sports* **2015**, 3(4), 312–324; doi: 10.3390/sports3040312
http://www.mdpi.com/2075-4663/3/4/312 20

Nathaniel D. M. Jenkins, Terry J. Housh, Samuel L. Buckner, Haley C. Bergstrom,
Kristen C. Cochrane, Cory M. Smith, Ethan C. Hill, Richard J. Schmidt and Joel T. Cramer
Individual Responses for Muscle Activation, Repetitions, and Volume during Three Sets to Failure
of High- (80% 1RM) *versus* Low-Load (30% 1RM) Forearm Flexion Resistance Exercise
Reprinted from: *Sports* **2015**, 3(4), 269–280; doi: 10.3390/sports3040269
http://www.mdpi.com/2075-4663/3/4/269 30

Nicole C. Dabbs, Jon A. Lundahl and John C. Garner
Effectiveness of Different Rest Intervals Following Whole-Body Vibration on Vertical Jump
Performance between College Athletes and Recreationally Trained Females
Reprinted from: *Sports* **2015**, 3(3), 258–268; doi: 10.3390/sports3030258
http://www.mdpi.com/2075-4663/3/3/258 40

Michael J. Duncan, Rosanna Gibbard, Leanne M. Raymond and Peter Mundy
The Effect of Kettlebell Swing Load and Cadence on Physiological, Perceptual and
Mechanical Variables
Reprinted from: *Sports* **2015**, 3(3), 202–208; doi: 10.3390/sports3030202
http://www.mdpi.com/2075-4663/3/3/202 49

Kristina M. Macias, Lee E. Brown, Jared W. Coburn and David D. Chen
A Comparison of Upper Body Strength between Rock Climbing and Resistance Trained Men
Reprinted from: *Sports* **2015**, 3(3), 178–187; doi: 10.3390/sports3030178
http://www.mdpi.com/2075-4663/3/3/178 55

Kevin A. Murach and James R. Bagley
Less Is More: The Physiological Basis for Tapering in Endurance, Strength, and Power Athletes
Reprinted from: *Sports* **2015**, 3(3), 209–218; doi: 10.3390/sports3030209
http://www.mdpi.com/2075-4663/3/3/209 63

Cassio V. Ruas, Ronei S. Pinto, Eduardo L. Cadore and Lee E. Brown
Angle Specific Analysis of Side-to-Side Asymmetry in the Shoulder Rotators
Reprinted from: *Sports* **2015**, *3*(3), 236–245; doi: 10.3390/sports3030236
http://www.mdpi.com/2075-4663/3/3/236 72

Isaiah T. McFarland, J. Jay Dawes, Craig L. Elder and Robert G. Lockie
Relationship of Two Vertical Jumping Tests to Sprint and Change of Direction Speed among Male
and Female Collegiate Soccer Players
Reprinted from: *Sports* **2016**, *4*(1), 11; doi: 10.3390/sports4010011
http://www.mdpi.com/2075-4663/4/1/11 80

Adebisi Bisi-Balogun and Firdevs Torlak
Outcomes following Hip and Quadriceps Strengthening Exercises for Patellofemoral Syndrome:
A Systematic Review and Meta-Analysis
Reprinted from: *Sports* **2015**, *3*(4), 281–301; doi: 10.3390/sports3040281
http://www.mdpi.com/2075-4663/3/4/281 87

About the Guest Editor

Lee Brown completed his graduate work and obtained his Ed.D. from Florida Atlantic University in Boca Raton, Florida. While a graduate assistant, he was responsible for isokinetic performance testing specifically designed to determine human responses to high velocity training. Dr. Brown joined the faculty at Cal State Fullerton in 2002 and is the current Director of the Center for Sport Performance and the Human Performance Laboratory. Prior to coming to California, he spent two years at Arkansas State University in Jonesboro, Arkansas as Director of the Human Performance Laboratory. Before Arkansas he was in Florida for 16 years serving as Research Director for an orthopedic surgeon's office and teaching and coaching at the public school level. He was President of the National Strength and Conditioning Association (NSCA), the NSCA Foundation and SWACSM. He currently sits on the Board of Trustees at National ACSM and is a Fellow of both the ACSM and the NSCA. His research interests include sport performance, anaerobic assessment and high velocity neuromuscular adaptations.

Preface to "Strength and Conditioning"

This Special Issue provides knowledge related to strength and conditioning for fitness and sport performance. It is designed for those interested in the many topics that concern strength and conditioning, in relation to advanced scientific inquiries of program design, periodization of training and anaerobic strength, and power testing. Topics focus on postactivation potentiation, neuromuscular adaptations to resistance training, motor unit recruitment, and muscle fiber types. Emphases are placed on investigations leading to increased human performance through manipulation of bioenergetics, biomechanics, and the endocrine system. Additionally, practical applications to training and performance are stressed, so as to influence daily exercise protocols.

Lee E. Brown
Guest Editor

![sports logo] *sports*

MDPI

Article

Lateral Squats Significantly Decrease Sprint Time in Collegiate Baseball Athletes

Jason B. White [1,†], Trevor P. Dorian [2,†] and Margaret T. Jones [1,*]

1   Health and Human Performance, George Mason University, Manassas, VA 20110, USA; jwhite35@gmu.edu
2   Exercise Science and Sport Studies, Springfield College, Springfield, MA 01109, USA
*   Correspondence: mjones15@gmu.edu; Tel.: +1-703-993-3247; Fax: +1-703-993-2025
†   These authors contributed equally to this work.

Academic Editor: Lee E. Brown
Received: 15 December 2015; Accepted: 1 March 2016; Published: 7 March 2016

Abstract: The purpose was to examine the effect of prior performance of dumbbell lateral squats (DBLS) on an agility movement-into-a-sprint (AMS) test. Twelve collegiate, resistance-trained, baseball athletes participated in three sessions separated by three days. Session One consisted of AMS baseline test, DBLS 5-RM test, and experimental protocol familiarization. Subjects were randomly assigned the protocol order for Sessions Two and Three, which consisted of warm up followed by 1-min sitting (no-DBLS) or performing the DBLS for 1×5 repetitions @ 5RM for each leg. Four minutes of slow recovery walking preceded the AMS test, which consisted of leading off a base and waiting for a visual stimulus. In reaction to stimulus, subjects exerted maximal effort while moving to the right by either pivoting or drop stepping and sprinting for 10 yards (yd). In Session Three, subjects switched protocols (DBLS, no-DBLS). Foot contact time (FCT), stride frequency (SF), stride length (SL), and 10-yd sprint time were measured. There were no differences between conditions for FCT, SF, or SL. Differences existed between DBLS (1.85 ± 0.09 s) and no-DBLS (1.89 ± 0.10 s) for AMS ($p = 0.03$). Results from the current study support the use of DBLS for performance enhancement prior to performing the AMS test.

Keywords: agility; complex training; lower body strength; postactivation potentiation; speed

1. Introduction

The importance of lower body muscular power to performance in sporting activities is well documented [1–3] Therefore, training techniques designed to improve lower body power are of interest, and methods such as plyometrics and complex training are commonly employed [4–6]. These training methods utilize exercises similar to the movements of sporting activity in order to provide sport specific enhancements and improve power development.

The response of skeletal muscle to specific stimuli is a function of the prior contraction history [7]. Complex training, a method that involves performing a moderate to heavy resistance exercise as a conditioning contraction followed by a lighter-resistance ballistic activity, has been shown to elicit greater lower body power production in subsequent explosive movements [8,9]. An example of complex training is performing a squat as the heavy strength exercise, followed by explosive vertical jumps. Acute performance enhancement found in power movements following a conditioning contraction exercise, such as a heavily loaded resistance exercise or maximal voluntary contractions (MVC), is likely due to post-activation potentiation (PAP) [10–14], which is defined as an increase in muscle function following a preload stimulus [7]. The application of complex training to elicit PAP, both acutely and in training programs, has long been thought to improve lower body power [4,15–17]. Both PAP and neuromuscular fatigue are stimulated by the same factors [18] and can occur simultaneously [19], but the greatest motor performance occurs with minimal neuromuscular fatigue [7]. It may be for this reason that the numerous studies that have examined complex training and PAP have pursued acute identification of the optimal load or the timing after loading where peak power production occurs. Previous research with resistance-trained athletes indicates that the optimal load for complex training may be achieved using MVCs [11] or 60%–85% 1-RM [20] and 3 to 8 min rest between the heavy strength exercise and the ensuing explosive movement [20,21]. However, the effect of complex training on PAP has been shown to vary with the individual's training status, exercise intensity, exercise volume, and length of rest period between the strength exercise and the explosive activity [20,22]. Further, it has been suggested that the interplay between a subject's individual characteristics and the protocol design (e.g., strength and power exercise selection) may have an important effect on the extent of potentiation elicited [23].

Strength is critical to developing force rapidly and is integral to the baseball skills of batting, throwing, and running [24], and agility movements (e.g., drop step, pivot, shuffle) are important when reacting to a stimulus (e.g., fielding, leading off of a base). Previous methodology to induce PAP has utilized dynamic movements, such as squat [13], bench press [25], Olympic lifts [26], loaded drop jumps [27], as well as isometric MVC [11,28]. Little research exists to indicate how PAP induced by lateral movements acutely impacts lower body power development. Further, because most studies have used the squat and vertical jump as the conditioning contraction exercise and ensuing explosive movement, respectively, little is known about the impact of loaded lateral strength exercises on explosive movement and power production. Yet, sports such as baseball, basketball, hockey, and football require as much as 50%–90% agility movements in a lateral direction [29]. Additionally, little research has been completed analyzing methods to improve the first stride in a frontal plane following a stationary athletic position. Therefore, the purpose of the current study was to examine the acute impact of dumbbell lateral squat (DBLS) exercise on an agility movement-into-a-sprint (AMS) test in collegiate baseball players.

2. Material and Methods

2.1. Subjects

Twelve (n = 12) National Collegiate Athletic Association (NCAA) Division-III resistance-trained baseball position players volunteered to participate in the current study. All subjects were proficient weight lifters and had $\geqslant$ 1 year of formal strength and conditioning training experience. All subjects were medically cleared for intercollegiate athletic participation, had the risks and benefits explained to them beforehand, signed an institutionally approved consent form to participate, and completed a medical history form. The Institutional Review Board for Human Subjects approved all procedures. Exclusion criteria consisted of severe musculoskeletal injuries of the lower body or spinal injuries within 6 months before the start of the study. The subjects were instructed to refrain from lower body exercise for 72 h before each testing session. Also, they were asked to consume an identical diet for the 24 h before each testing session. Testing sessions were conducted during the off-season training period. All subjects in the current study were members of the same baseball team, and were familiar with the DBLS exercise and the AMS test from their participation in the same collegiate strength and conditioning off-season program. Physical characteristics are included in Table 1.

Table 1. Physical characteristics of baseball athletes.

Physical Characteristic	Mean	SD
Age (y)	19.9	1.2
Training experience (y)	3.2	2.1
Height (cm)	175.9	6.6
Body mass (kg)	79.9	10.9
5-RM DBLS (kg)	18.2	4.9

n = 12. Year (y); Centimeter (cm); Kilogram (kg); Standard deviation (*SD*).

2.2. Experimental Design

The purpose of the current study was to investigate the acute effect of DBLS exercise on an agility movement into a 10 yd sprint. A within-subject randomized crossover design was used as subjects completed the AMS test following DBLS exercise and a control condition (no-DBLS) without DBLS exercise. In both the DBLS and no-DBLS conditions, four minutes of slow recovery walking preceded the AMS test.

2.3. Procedures

2.3.1. Session One: 5-RM DBLS Testing and Protocol Familiarization

Session One consisted of completing the informed consent and medical history forms, familiarization with the 10-min supervised standardized warm-up (*i.e.*, five minutes of stationary cycling at 70–80 RPM with a 0.5-kg load and five min of dynamic flexibility exercises), application of reflective markers, baseline AMS test, and 5-RM DBLS test. Prior to testing and familiarization, subjects' height and body mass were determined to the nearest 0.1 cm and 0.1 kg, respectively, using a stadiometer (Tanita; Arlington Heights, IL, USA) and self-calibrating digital scale (Tanita; Arlington Heights, IL, USA) with subjects in sock feet.

2.3.2. Sessions Two and Three: Experimental Protocol

Seventy-two hours after Session One, subjects returned to the laboratory at the same time of day on two separate occasions, each separated by seventy-two hours, to perform two randomly ordered experimental trials (DBLS, no-DBLS). Athletes were randomly assigned to the DBLS or no-DBLS protocol. In Session Three, which took place 72 h later, the subjects switched protocols. On the day of each experimental trial, subjects arrived having refrained from lower body resistive exercise since the previous experimental trial. After a supervised, standardized, 10-min warm-up identical to that performed prior to testing during session one, subjects performed DBLS exercise of 1×5 repetitions @ 5-RM for each leg or sat quietly for 1 min, depending upon their assigned protocol. The DBLS exercise was performed according to the methods described for the 5-RM test. However, both legs were trained. After the left knee flexed to meet the proper squat depth five consecutive times, the right leg followed. Following four minutes of slow recovery walking subjects performed the AMS test.

2.3.3. 5-RM DBLS Test

Lateral squat [30] strength was assessed for the right leg with a 5-RM test using dumbbells. Briefly, subjects completed a 10-min whole body warm up followed by supervised warm up sets for the DBLS test. While performing the DBLS, the athlete assumed a stance approximately twice that of shoulder width (Figure 1). Each subject's foot placement was measured and recorded. The pelvis was tilted posteriorly and the subject performed a downward squatting motion until the anterior thigh was parallel to the floor. When the subject reached parallel squat depth, a sound was emitted from the safety squat beeper (Bigger, Faster, Stronger, Inc., Salt Lake City, UT, USA), which had been placed anteriorly on the thigh of the right leg [24]. The beeper location was noted for each subject and repeated for subsequent experimental sessions. In the down position of the DBLS, both heels remained in contact with the floor. The down position was held for one second. Upon completion of the down position, the subject rose to the upward position with full extension in the hips and knees, while keeping the feet in contact with ground. Dumbbells were rested upon the anterior deltoids of the subject in a front squat hold position. A timed rest of three minutes was taken before each maximal effort set. Weight was increased based upon the performance of the previous attempt, and the subject continued to perform sets of five repetitions until failure or until it was determined that he could no longer perform the DBLS safely with proper form. After two failures, testing was stopped, and the best lift for 5-RM was recorded.

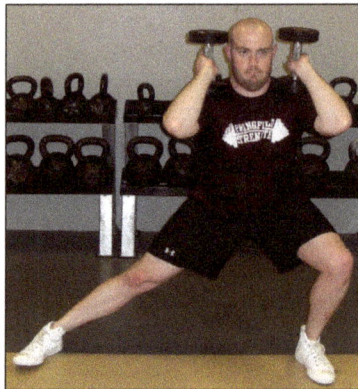

Figure 1. Mid-range of the DBLS exercise.

2.3.4. AMS Test

The AMS test was conducted in the laboratory following the DBLS or no-DBLS exercise. All subjects performed a 4-min slow walking recovery [21] prior to the start of the AMS test. The AMS consisted of performing a 10-yd sprint from a base runner's stance for the starting position. Ten reflective markers were applied to the body: left and right anterior superior iliac spine, center of the left and right patella, left and right mid-thigh, distal anterior portion of the left and right tibia, medial malleolus on the right leg, and lateral malleolus on the left leg. Individual anatomical locations of marker placements were located and marked on each subject with semi-permanent ink to enable reproducibility for subsequent measures. Athletes were required to wear compression shorts to clarify movement of the lower extremities for the video analysis. Prior to the initiation of the agility movement, the subject was stationary and had a stance slightly wider than shoulder width, with slight flexion in the knees and hips. Body weight was distributed evenly on the balls of the feet, and both feet were parallel with the sagittal plane. Each subject's foot placement was measured and recorded. The direction of movement was to the right of the subject in the frontal plane, which is identical to stealing a base in baseball; consequently, athletes were well versed in the movement. The initial movement began upon reaction to a visual stimulus, which was a light emitting diode. The subject exerted maximal effort while moving to the right by either pivoting both feet or drop stepping with the right foot in order to place the feet in a position similar to that of a linear sprint during initial acceleration. The subject maximally sprinted for 10 yd. Each athlete's choice of a pivot or drop step was noted by the researcher and repeated during subsequent testing sessions.

In AMS testing Sessions Two and Three, the foot contact time (FCT) and stride length (SL) for the Stride 1 and Stride 2, and stride frequency (SF) for Segment 1 and Segment 2 were recorded by a video camera (50 fps, JVC GR-DVL9800 Mini, JVC USA, Wayne, NJ), which was placed perpendicular to the sagittal plane of the subject and 10 yd from the running lane. Markers were placed at 0, 5, and 10 yd on the blank wall that was parallel to the running lane. The same trained researcher analyzed all recordings using two-dimensional video analysis software (Dartfish 5.0 Connect, Fribourg, Switzerland). Timing sensors with single beamed infrared photocells (Brower Timing Systems, Salt Lake City, UT, USA) were placed to capture the time at the 5 and 10 yd locations.

Test-retest reliability for the AMS was determined from data collected during baseline AMS tests in session one and the subsequent no-DBLS condition, which was either Session Two or Three depending upon the random order assignment of each subject's no-DBLS condition.

Foot contact time (FCT). The FCT time was defined as the time that each foot was in contact with the ground following initial lower body movement. The initial movement pattern varied based upon how the athletes were taught to steal a base (*i.e.*, drop step *vs.* pivot). Approximately half of the athletes drop stepped with the right foot prior to pivoting and striding with the left. Only FCT prior to a stride was recorded in order to maintain consistency among measures. Athletes repeated their chosen initial movement (*i.e.*, drop step, pivot) for both DBLS and no-DBLS conditions.

Stride frequency (SF). For comparison of SF or number of strides per section of distance, the AMS test was divided into two segments: 0–5 (Segment 1) and 6–10 yd (Segment 2). Using video analysis, SF for each segment was determined from the total number of strides taken during the total time taken to cover Segment 1 and to cover Segment 2.

Stride length (SL). Stride length for Stride 1 and Stride 2 were determined from video analysis and recorded in inches for both experimental sessions. Stride 1 was defined as the distance covered between first two successive ground contacts by the left foot. Stride 2 was defined as the distance covered between next two successive ground contacts by the right foot.

2.4. Statistical Analyses

Normality of data was assessed by the Kolmogorov-Smirnov test of normality, which determined all primary outcome measures of interest to be normally distributed. Foot contact (FCT), stride frequency (SF), and stride length (SL) were analyzed with 2 (condition: DBLS, no-DBLS) × 2 [time (FCT), distance (SL), number (SF)] repeated measures analysis of variance (ANOVA). The AMS test was analyzed by a 2 (condition) × 3 (segment 1, segment 2, total time) repeated measures ANOVA. Bonferroni's pairwise post hoc analyses examined differences across condition and within testing periods. Effect sizes were calculated and a modified classification system (trivial, 0.0–0.2; small, 0.2–0.6; moderate, 0.6–1.2; large, 1.2–2.0; very large, >2.0; extremely large, >4.0) was used [31]. Test-retest reliability was determined through the intra-class correlation coefficient (ICC). Statistical procedures were conducted using the Statistical Package for the Social Sciences (IBM SPSS Statistics 20.0, IBM Corporation, Armonk, NY, USA). The alpha level was set at $p < 0.05$.

3. Results

There was no significant interaction between the DBLS and no-DBLS conditions for FCT ($p = 0.70$), SF ($p = 0.28$), or SL ($p = 0.79$) (Table 2). Significant differences were found for FCT (ES = 5.3, $p = 0.0001$) and SL (ES = 1.2, $p = 0.0004$) between Stride 1 and Stride 2. The SF for Segment 2 (6–10 yard) was significantly (ES = 2.2, $p < 0.0002$) less than for Segment 1 (0–5 yard). A significant difference existed between conditions for the AMS test for Segment 1 time (ES = 0.61, $p = 0.01$, DBLS: 1.11 ± 0.06 s; no-DBLS: 1.15 ± 0.07 s), and total time (ES = 0.42, $p = 0.03$, DBLS: 1.85 ± 0.09 s; no-DBLS: 1.89 ± 0.10 s) (Figure 2). There was no significant difference ($p = 0.414$) in overall AMS time between session one (1.90 ± 0.09 s) and the no-DBLS condition (1.89 ± 0.10 s), and the ICC of 0.98 between the two testing sessions was considered strong.

Table 2. Foot contact, stride frequency, and stride length for DBLS and no-DBLS conditions.

Measure	DBLS Condition M ± SD	no-DBLS Condition M ± SD
Foot Contact Time (FCT) (s):		
Stride 1	0.39 ± 0.05	0.38 ± 0.04
Stride 2	0.64 ± 0.04 *	0.63 ± 0.06 *
Stride Frequency (SF):		
0–5 yd (Segment 1)	3.75 ± 0.45	3.75 ± 0.45
6–10 yd (Segment 2)	2.92 ± 0.29 #	2.67 ± 0.49 #
Stride Length (SL) (in):		
Stride 1	46.52 ± 3.97	46.19 ± 5.75
Stride 2	52.23 ± 5.36 *	51.54 ± 7.11 *

* Significant difference ($p < 0.001$) between Stride 1 and Stride 2; # significant difference ($p < 0.001$) between 0 and 5 yd (Segment 1) and 6 and 10 yd (Segment 2); n = 12, yd (yard), s (second), in (inch).

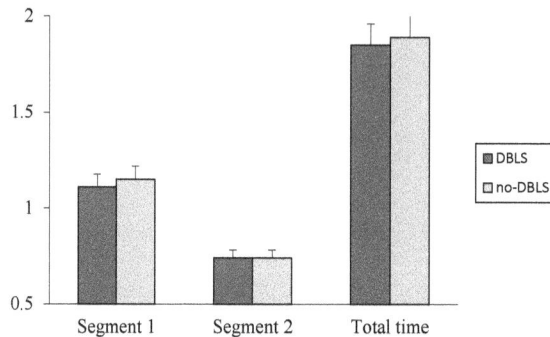

Figure 2. AMS test time (s) for DBLS and no-DBLS conditions. [#] significant difference ($p < 0.05$) between total LMS time for DBLS and no-DBLS conditions; * significant difference ($p < 0.05$) between Segment 1 (0–5 yd) and Segment 2 (6–10 yd).

4. Discussion

This is the first study to examine whether or not an acute bout of DBLS exercise would enhance agility movement and the subsequent sprint in resistance-trained, collegiate baseball athletes. It was hypothesized that measures of FCT, SF, SL, and AMS time would improve as a result of acute lower body resistive exercise. The overall findings supported a positive effect on the use of resistive exercise on AMS time; however, no difference was found for FCT, SF, or SL across the DBLS and no-DBLS conditions. To our knowledge, no study to date has reported on the effect of complex training on an agility movement-into-a-sprint, FCT, SF, or SL in baseball athletes, yet, baseball is a sport that requires a large percentage of agility movements in a lateral direction [29]. The performance measure (AMS test) in the current study was comparable to the baseball specific movement of stealing a base [32]. It required reaction to a visual stimulus, quick change of direction, and a short burst sprint, all of which are regularly used movement patterns in baseball [33].

The mechanisms responsible for eliciting PAP and the optimal conditions for performance enhancement from complex training have not been clearly defined. The utilization of dynamic strength movements for a conditioning exercise to induce PAP during plyometric exercise has yielded mixed results [10,14,23,34–36]. Previous research has demonstrated improved sprint times following single joint and isometric strength exercise [37]. However, the effect of dynamic strength exercise on sprint time is equivocal and varies by individual and rest time [21,22]. Further, the exercise selection and intensity of the conditioning contraction can impact subsequent power production [20]. Complex training has resulted in improved 10-m shuttle run time [38], 10-m [22], 40-m [13], and 100-m [39] sprint times. In contrast, other research has shown no effect on 10-m [13], 30-m [24] and 40-m [26] sprint times.

In the current study, complex training did not elicit a PAP response for the FCT, which was defined as the time that each foot was in contact with the ground following initial lower body movement until the foot completed the stride. The contact time for Stride 1 was significantly lower than Stride 2, irrespective of DBLS or no-DBLS condition. This was likely due to the required movement direction to the right, which was similar to that necessary when stealing a base. As a result, the left foot always completed Stride 1, and the right foot stayed in contact with the ground for a longer period of time. Varying differences in the agility movement patterns (drop step, pivot) were existent, but not the focus of the current study.

Complex training did not elicit a PAP response for the SF. In both conditions the SF for Segment 1 was significantly greater than Segment 2, which is likely a result of the short explosive strides required during the initial acceleration of Segment 1 *versus* the longer strides of Segment 2 as the athlete increased his running speed [40].

The primary purpose of examining SL was to determine change in SL due to PAP; however, the condition (DBLS, no-DBLS) had no effect on SL in the current study. Irrespective of condition, Stride 2 was significantly greater than Stride 1, and this finding was likely due to the specific mechanical tendencies of the movement pattern. The initial agility movement that was performed prior to sprinting was identical to that of a baseball player attempting to steal a base; therefore, the subject was required to move to his right in the frontal plane following a stationary athletic position. After visual examination of the digital recordings of running mechanics it was clear that an initial stride of the subject with the left foot was needed in order to rotate the hips and shoulders to the right and rapidly move the center of gravity so that the momentum of the subject was correctly oriented toward the target. The pivoting limited the initial stride of the left foot. The subject could then make a significantly greater second stride with the left foot because he was facing in the direction of the sprinting destination.

Regardless of condition (DBLS, no-DBLS) the AMS test time for Segment 2 (6–10 yd) was significantly lower than Segment 1 (0–5 yd), which is likely a result of the athlete beginning the AMS test from a stationary athletic stance position. After accelerating through the 5 yd sensor and completing Segment 1, the athlete had created enough momentum to propel himself through Segment 2 and the final 10 yd sensor at a faster speed.

While FCT, SL, and SF, did not differ between DBLS and no-DBLS conditions, AMS Segment 1 and total time were significantly lower (0.04 s) for the DBLS condition than the no-DBLS condition; therefore, the resistive exercise may have induced PAP, which enhanced the sprint time. Segment 1 was 3.6% faster and the total AMS time was 2.2% faster when the AMS was preceded by DBLS. Although the effect size was small, milliseconds can determine whether or not a base runner is safe or out, therefore, such a magnitude of improvement might have noteworthy ramifications during competition. In the current study, the DBLS exercise was followed by a 4-min rest period during which the subjects completed a slow recovery walk prior to performing the AMS test. In previous research reporting a significant PAP effect during sprinting distances of 10-m [22], 30-m [38], 40-m [13], and 100-m [39], the dynamic resistance exercise selection and intensity have varied for the conditioning contraction, but the most effective rest periods have consistently been $\geqslant$ 4 min. The design of the current study was unique because it examined the effects of PAP on a ballistic agility movement that led into a sprint. The use of resistance-trained baseball athletes who were familiar with the AMS test and the DBLS in conjunction with the standardization of all warm-up procedures may have also been contributing factors in the positive results of the current study.

We acknowledge some study limitations. First, although all subjects in the current study were resistance-trained collegiate baseball position players, the sample size of twelve was small. A larger sample size may have resulted in other differences between the DBLS and no-DBLS conditions. It has been demonstrated that results from studies examining PAP in relation to performance on field tests are equivocal, in part due to the varied individual response to complex training methods [20,22,26]. Second, a higher grade of video analysis software may have allowed for better discrimination in measures of FCT, SL, and SF.

It is well known that responses to a PAP protocol may vary depending upon the individual's training background and strength level [14,23,34,36,39]. Future research that examines the effects of dynamic strength movements on varied sprint distances, repeated sprint measures, and the establishment of how long the PAP effect remains are warranted. The investigation of efficiency of various agility movement patterns (e.g., drop step, pivot) for directional change would also be of interest. Further, the effect of implementing such complex training methods between innings during game play would be of interest to the baseball practitioner.

5. Conclusions

Results from the current study are applicable to sport and training. Successful skill execution in baseball often requires the development of power over a short period of time. Effective use of

PAP (movement specific conditioning exercise, proper rest time) in the form of complex training can enable an individual to train at a greater intensity, therefore, attaining superior gains in power production. Program implementation of complex training, which pairs DB lateral squats with short sprints, may provide an adequate training stimulus for enhancing agility movements and, thereby, improve base running.

Acknowledgments: The authors would like to thank the athletic trainers, coaches, and student-athletes from the intercollegiate baseball program, for their contribution to the study.

Author Contributions: All authors were involved in study design, data collection, data interpretation, and manuscript writing.

Conflicts of Interest: The authors declare no conflict of interest.

References

1. Baker, D.; Nance, S. The relation between strength and power in professional rugby league players. *J. Strength Cond. Res.* **1999**, *13*, 224–229. [CrossRef]
2. Hawley, J.A.; Williams, M.M.; Vickovic, M.M.; Handcock, P.J. Muscle power predicts freestyle swimming performance. *Br. J. Sport Med.* **1992**, *26*, 151–155. [CrossRef]
3. Silvestre, R.; West, C.; Maresh, C.M.; Kraemer, W.J. Body composition and physical performance in men's soccer: A study of a national collegiate athletic association division I team. *J. Strength Cond. Res.* **2007**, *20*, 177–183. [CrossRef] [PubMed]
4. Bauer, T.; Thayer, R.E.; Baras, G. Comparison of training modalities for power development in the lower extremity. *J. Strength Cond. Res.* **1990**, *4*, 115–121. [CrossRef]
5. Dodd, D.J.; Alvar, B.A. Analysis of acute explosive training modalities to improve lower-body power in baseball players. *J. Strength Cond. Res.* **2007**, *21*, 1177–1182. [CrossRef] [PubMed]
6. Potteiger, J.A.; Lockwood, R.H.; Haub, M.D.; Dolezal, B.A.; Almuzaini, K.S.; Schroeder, J.M.; Zebas, C.J. Muscle power and fiber characteristics following 8 weeks of plyometric training. *J. Strength Cond. Res.* **1999**, *13*, 275–279. [CrossRef]
7. Hodgson, M.; Docherty, D.; Robbins, D. Post-activation potentiation underlying physiology and implications for motor performance. *Sports Med.* **2005**, *35*, 585–595. [CrossRef] [PubMed]
8. Chiu, L.Z.; Fry, A.C.; Weiss, L.W.; Schilling, B.K.; Brown, L.E.; Smith, S.L. Postactivation potentiation response in athletic and recreationally trained individuals. *J. Strength Cond. Res.* **2003**, *17*, 671–677. [CrossRef] [PubMed]
9. Tillin, M.N.A.; Bishop, D. Factors modulating post-activation potentiation and its effect on performance of subsequent explosive activities. *Sports Med.* **2009**, *39*, 147–166. [CrossRef] [PubMed]
10. Baker, D. Acute effect of alternating heavy and light resistance on power output during upper-body complex power training. *J. Strength Cond. Res.* **2003**, *17*, 493–497. [CrossRef] [PubMed]
11. Gullich, A.; Schmidtbleicher, D. MVC-induced short-term potentiation of explosive force. *New Stud. Athlet.* **1996**, *11*, 67–81.
12. Hamada, T.; Sale, D.G.; Macdougall, J.D.; Tarnopolsky, M.A. Postactivation potentiation, fiber type, and twitch contraction time in human knee extensor muscles. *J. Appl. Physiol.* **2000**, *88*, 2131–2144. [PubMed]
13. McBride, J.; Nimphius, S.; Erickson, T.M. The acute effects of heavy-load squats and loaded countermovement jumps on sprint performance. *J. Strength Cond. Res.* **2005**, *19*, 893–897. [CrossRef] [PubMed]
14. Young, W.B.; Jenner, A.; Griffiths, K. Acute enhancement of power performance from heavy load squats. *J. Strength Cond. Res.* **1998**, *12*, 82–84. [CrossRef]
15. Adams, K.; O'Shea, J.P.; O'Shea, K.L.; Climstein, M. The effect of six weeks of squat, plyometric and squat-plyometric training on power production. *J. Strength Cond. Res.* **1992**, *6*, 36–41. [CrossRef]
16. Ebben, W.P.; Watts, P.B. A review of combined weight training and plyometric training modes: Complex training. *Strength Cond. J.* **1998**, *20*, 18–27. [CrossRef]
17. Verkhoshansky, Y.; Tetyan, V. Speed-strength preparation of future champions. *Legk. Athlet.* **1973**, *2*, 12–13.
18. Rassier, D.; Herzog, W. The effects of training on fatigue and twitch potentiation in human skeletal muscle. *Eur. J. Sport Sci.* **2001**, *1*, 177–192. [CrossRef]

19. Rassier, D.E.; MacIntosh, B.R. Coexistence of potentiation and fatigue in skeletal muscle. *Braz. J. Med. Biol. Res.* **2000**, *30*, 499–508. [CrossRef]

20. Wilson, J.M.; Duncan, N.M.; Marin, P.J.; Brown, L.E.; Loenneke, J.P.; Wilson, S.M.C.; Jo, E.; Lowery, R.P.; Ugrinowitsch, C. Meta-analysis of postactivation potentiation and power: Effects of conditioning activity, volume, gender, rest periods, and training status. *J. Strength Cond. Res.* **2013**, *27*, 854–859. [CrossRef] [PubMed]

21. Comyns, T.M.; Harrison, A.J.; Hennessy, L.K.; Jensen, R.L. The optimal complex training rest interval for athletes from anaerobic sports. *J. Strength Cond. Res.* **2006**, *20*, 471–476. [CrossRef] [PubMed]

22. Bevan, H.R.; Cunningham, D.J.; Tooley, E.P.; Owen, N.J.; Cook, C.J.; Kilduff, L.P. Influence of postactivation potentiation on sprinting performance in professional rugby players. *J. Strength Cond. Res.* **2010**, *24*, 701–705. [CrossRef] [PubMed]

23. Suchomel, T.J.; Lamont, H.S.; Moir, G.L. Understanding vertical jump potentiation: A deterministic model. *Sports Med.* **2015**. [CrossRef] [PubMed]

24. Jones, M.T. Effect of compensatory acceleration training in combination with accommodating resistance on upper body strength in collegiate athletes. *Open Access J. Sports Med.* **2014**, *5*, 183–189. [CrossRef] [PubMed]

25. Hrysomallis, D.; Kidgell, D. Effect of heavy dynamic resistive exercise on acute upper-body power. *J. Strength Cond. Res.* **2001**, *15*, 426–430. [CrossRef] [PubMed]

26. Guggenheimer, J.D.; Dickin, D.C.; Reyes, G.F.; Dolny, D.G. The effects of specific preconditioning activities on acute sprint performance. *J. Strength Cond. Res.* **2009**, *23*, 1135–1139. [CrossRef] [PubMed]

27. Lima, J.B.; Marin, D.P.; Barquilha, G.; Da Silva, L.O.; Puggina, E.F.; Pithon-Curi, T.C.; Hirabarai, S.M. Acute effects of drop jump potentiation protocol on sprint and counter movement vertical jump performance. *Hum. Mov. Sci.* **2011**, *12*, 324–330.

28. Lim, J.H.; Kong, P.W. Effects of isometric and dynamic postactivation potentiation protocols on maximal sprint performance. *J. Strength Cond. Res.* **2013**, *27*, 2730–2736. [CrossRef] [PubMed]

29. MacClean, C.R. Sport-specific and lateral conditioning. *Scholast. Coach* **1993**, 14–17.

30. Hedrick, A. Using free weights to improve lateral movement performance. *Strength Cond. J.* **1999**, *21*, 21–25. [CrossRef]

31. Hopkins, W.; Marshall, S.; Batterham, A.; Hanin, J. Progressive statistics for studies in sports medicine and exercise science. *Med. Sci. Sports Exerc.* **2009**, *41*, 3–12. [CrossRef] [PubMed]

32. Caliendo, P. *Youth Baseball Drills*, 1st ed.; Human Kinetics: Champaign, IL, USA, 2014; pp. 134–151.

33. Priest, J.W.; Jones, J.N.; Conger, B.; Marble, D.K. Performance measures of NCAA baseball tryouts obtained from the new 60-yd run-shuttle. *J. Strength Cond. Res.* **2011**, *25*, 2872–2878. [CrossRef] [PubMed]

34. Duthie, G.M.; Young, W.B.; Aitken, D.A. The acute effects of heavy loads on jump squat performance: An evaluation of the complex and contrast methods of power development. *J. Strength Cond. Res.* **2002**, *16*, 530–538. [CrossRef] [PubMed]

35. Gourgoulis, V.; Aggeloussis, N.; Kasimatis, P.; Mavromatis, G.; Garas, A. Effect of a submaximal half-squats warm-up program on vertical jumping ability. *J. Strength Cond. Res.* **2003**, *17*, 342–344. [CrossRef] [PubMed]

36. Rixon, K.P.; Lamont, H.S.; Bemben, M.G. Influence of type of muscle contraction, gender, and lifting experience on postactivation potentiation performance. *J. Strength Cond. Res.* **2007**, *21*, 500–505. [CrossRef] [PubMed]

37. Sale, D.G. Postactivation potentiation: Role in human performance. *Exerc. Sport Sci. Rev.* **2002**, *30*, 138–143. [CrossRef] [PubMed]

38. Okuno, N.M.; Tricoli, V.; Silva, S.B.C.; Bertuzzi, R.; Moreira, A.; Kiss, M.A.P.D.M. Postactivation potentiation on repeated-sprint ability in elite handball players. *J. Strength Cond. Res.* **2013**, *27*, 662–668. [CrossRef] [PubMed]

39. Linder, E.E.; Prins, J.H.; Murata, N.M.; Derenne, C.; Morgan, C.F.; Solomon, J.R. Effects of preload 4 repetition maximum on 100-m sprint times in collegiate women. *J. Strength Cond. Res.* **2010**, *24*, 1184–1190. [CrossRef] [PubMed]

40. Plisk, S. Speed, agility and speed-endurance development. In *Essentials of Strength Training and Conditioning*, 3rd ed.; Baechle, T.R., Earle, R.W., Eds.; Human Kinetics: Champaign, IL, USA, 2008; pp. 457–485.

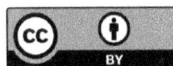

![sports logo] *sports*

[MDPI]

Article

Effects of Short-Term Dynamic Constant External Resistance Training and Subsequent Detraining on Strength of the Trained and Untrained Limbs: A Randomized Trial

Pablo B. Costa [1,*], Trent J. Herda [2,†], Ashley A. Herda [2,†] and Joel T. Cramer [3]

[1]   Exercise Physiology Laboratory, Department of Kinesiology, California State University, Fullerton,
      CA 92831, USA
[2]   Department of Health, Sport and Exercise Sciences, University of Kansas, Lawrence, KS 66045, USA;
      t.herda@ku.edu (T.J.H.); a.herda@ku.edu (A.A.H.)
[3]   Department of Nutrition and Health Sciences, University of Nebraska—Lincoln, Lincoln, NE 68583, USA;
      jcramer@unl.edu
*   Correspondence: pcosta@fullerton.edu; Tel.: +1-657-278-4232; Fax: +1-657-278-2103
†   These authors contributed equally to this work.

Academic Editor: Eling de Bruin
Received: 14 December 2015; Accepted: 25 January 2016; Published: 27 January 2016

Abstract: Short-term resistance training has been shown to increase isokinetic muscle strength and performance after only two to nine days of training. The purpose of this study was to examine the effects of three days of unilateral dynamic constant external resistance (DCER) training and detraining on the strength of the trained and untrained legs. Nineteen men were randomly assigned to a DCER training group or a non-training control group. Subjects visited the laboratory eight times, the first visit was a familiarization session, the second visit was a pre-training assessment, the subsequent three visits were for training sessions (if assigned to the training group), and the last three visits were post-training assessments 1, 2, and 3 (*i.e.*, 48 h, 1 week, and 2 weeks after the final training session). Strength increased in both trained and untrained limbs from pre- to post-training assessment 1 for the training group and remained elevated at post-training assessments 2 and 3 ($p \leq 0.05$). No changes were observed in the control ($p > 0.05$). Possible strength gains from short-term resistance training have important implications in clinical rehabilitation settings, sports injury prevention, as well as other allied health fields such as physical therapy, occupational therapy, and athletic training.

Keywords: training-induced; neuromuscular adaptation; isotonic; muscle mechanics; unilateral; cross education

1. Introduction

Allied health professionals, such as physical therapists, occupational therapists, and athletic trainers, may benefit from rapid increases in strength of a patient or athlete recovering from injury [1–3]. In theory, if an individual's strength can be increased within a short period of time, an alternative to more expensive and invasive medical procedures may be offered [1,2]. In addition, they are more likely to comply with a rehabilitation program and perhaps decrease the risk of reinjury [3]. Consequently, short-term resistance training has been shown to increase isokinetic muscle strength and performance after only two to nine days of training [1,2,4,5]. This short time course for strength adaptations may conveniently coincide with the commonly limited rehabilitation treatments due to minimal insurance coverage or lack of compliance [1,2], or the time demands for return to play in sports. If patients do not improve quickly, the risk of injury reoccurrence may increase [1]. This potential for short-term resistance training to improve muscular performance in a relatively shorter period of time would have important implications for professionals working in rehabilitation settings [1–3].

Evidence has shown that improvements in muscle performance can be observed in a shorter period than what is typically used in longer traditional training programs [1,2,6,7]. For example, Prevost *et al.*, (1999) investigated velocity-specific short-term training for two days and reported 22.1% increases in peak torque (PT) at $270°·s^{-1}$ after training at $270°·s^{-1}$, but no changes for training at 30 and $150°·s^{-1}$ at the testing velocities of 30 and $150°·s^{-1}$ [4]. Similarly, Coburn *et al.*, (2006) compared short-term resistance training effects after three sessions of slow- or fast-velocity and found that PT increased for both training groups [2]. However, the slower velocity training group increased PT at both velocities whereas PT increased only at the faster velocity for the faster velocity training group [2]. No changes in PT were observed for the control group and no changes in EMG amplitude were reported for any of the groups at any of the velocities. The authors concluded three sessions of slow or fast velocity isokinetic resistance training were sufficient to increase PT and the lack of EMG amplitude changes suggested increases in leg extension PT were not caused by increases in muscle activation [2].

The principle of training called reversibility, or detraining, occurs when a complete cessation or substantial reduction in training causes a partial or complete reversal of the adaptations induced by training [8,9]. Detraining occurs after an individual discontinues a training program [8–15]. Most of the increases in strength found with resistance training are lost after several weeks of detraining [10–14,16,17]. However, Colliander and Tesch (1992) showed that a resistance training program incorporating combined concentric and eccentric leg extension exercise retained more of the novel strength gains than a concentric-only training program [16]. In addition, Farthing (2003) found eccentric muscle action training elicited greater strength gains than concentric training [18]. Because isokinetic muscle actions are typically concentric, it is unknown whether dynamic constant external resistance (DCER) training, which uses coupled concentric and eccentric muscle actions, and isokinetic training would affect detraining differently.

Isokinetic muscle actions have been traditionally used in rehabilitation and testing scenarios. Several studies have examined the effects of isokinetic training on strength and/or muscle cross-sectional area (CSA) [1,2,4,5] and isokinetic training allows development of maximum tension throughout the range of motion [7]. However, DCER training would offer a more accessible, convenient, cost-effective, and practical method of training, in addition to perhaps providing a greater stimulus to elicit increases in strength [19]. Furthermore, no studies have investigated the effects of short term resistance training on the contralateral untrained limb or on detraining. Therefore, the purpose of this study was to examine the effects of three days of DCER training and subsequent detraining on isokinetic on strength of the trained and untrained contralateral leg extensors during maximal leg extension muscle actions.

2. Method

2.1. Subjects

Nineteen apparently healthy untrained men (mean ± SD age = 21.6 ± 3.4 years; body mass = 77.9 ± 14.0 kg; height = 173.9 ± 4.1 cm) were randomly assigned to a DCER training group or control group. Participants were minimally active and naïve to the intent of the study. Individuals with a history of chronic resistance training (>1 day/week) in the previous 12 months or those who reported engaging in one or more lower-body resistance training exercise for six months prior to the start of the study were excluded from participating. Prior to any testing, all subjects read and signed an informed consent form and completed a health status questionnaire. Individuals with any degenerative neuromuscular or joint disorders, or who sustained injuries distal to the waist within six months prior to screening were also excluded from the study. Subjects were asked to maintain their daily activities, but refrain from any exercise and/or nutritional supplements throughout the course of the study. Individuals who had been taking nutritional supplements three months prior to screening were not permitted to participate. This study was approved by the university's Institutional Review Board for the Protection of Human Subjects.

2.2. Research Design

A mixed factorial design was used to examine the effects of three days of short-term unilateral resistance training and subsequent detraining on strength. Subjects visited the laboratory on eight separate occasions. The first visit was a familiarization session, the second visit was a pre-training assessment, the subsequent three visits were for training (if assigned to the training group), and the last three visits were the post-training assessments (*i.e.*, 48 h, 1 week, and 2 weeks after the final training session). Pre-training assessments were performed 48 h prior to the start of training. Testing included assessments of DCER strength. The training group performed DCER leg extension exercise with the dominant leg in each of the three days of training whereas the control group did not take part in the training intervention. After the three training sessions, post-training assessments were performed in an identical manner to the pre-training assessments. In order to examine the time course of the effects of training, post-training assessments were performed 48 h, 1 week, and 2 weeks after the final training session. All pre- and post-training assessments were conducted at approximately the same time of day.

2.3. Dynamic Constant External Resistance Assessments

The maximal strength of the leg extensors were assessed using a DCER Nautilus leg extension machine (Nautilus, Inc., Vancouver, WA, USA). The input axis of the machine was aligned with the axis of rotation of the knee. The distal anterior portion of the leg superior to the ankle was used as the load bearing point. Three submaximal warm-up sets of increasing tester-selected intensities (*i.e.*, 6–8, 3–5, and 1–2 repetitions) preceded the maximal strength attempt. When one attempt was successful, the load was increased by 2–5 kg until a failed repetition occurred. A failed repetition was defined as the inability to complete the full range of motion with the assigned load. During the tests, loud verbal encouragement was provided by the investigator. Each subject was instructed to provide maximal effort throughout the entire range of motion. The greatest load moved through a complete leg extension range of motion was considered the one repetition maximum (1-RM). A 1-min rest was allowed between each successive attempt [20,21].

2.4. Dynamic Constant External Resistance Training Protocol

After a rest period of 48 h following the pre-training assessment, the training group took part in three DCER training sessions separated by 48 h. Participants in the training group performed 4 sets of 10 repetitions. Each training session began with ten warm-up repetitions at approximately 25% of the resistance used for the DCER training session. Approximately 80% of the 1-RM obtained during the DCER maximal strength assessment was used as the starting load for the DCER group. A 2-min rest period was allowed between each training set. Training load for the DCER group was continually increased and adjusted by approximately 1.14 kg as each participant was able to tolerate a given load with ease in order to ensure that the subject reached failure at approximately the 10th repetition. All participants taking part in the DCER training intervention were supervised during all training sessions.

2.5. Rating of Perceived Exertion

Rating of perceived exertion (RPE) was used to compare effort among the DCER training days and sets [22–26]. Prior to the start of the study, subjects received instructions on how to use the RPE scale to rate their perceived exertion. A Category-Ratio scale (CR-10) was used, where "0" is classified as rest (no effort) and "10" is classified as maximal effort (most stressful exercise ever performed). The CR-10 has been slightly modified to reflect American English (e.g., easy and hard instead of light and strong, respectively) [24]. Subjects were asked to provide a number on the scale to rate their overall effort immediately after each set was completed and after the entire training session. The RPE assessments were conducted during each session by showing the scale and asking subjects "How would you rate your effort?" and "How would you rate your entire workout?" immediately after each set of training and after each training session, respectively. Therefore, in this study, "set RPE" was defined as the RPE reported by the subject after each set, while "session RPE" was defined as the RPE reported each day after the training session was completed.

2.6. Statistical Analyses

A three-way mixed factorial ANOVA (time (pre- *vs.* post-training assessment 1 *vs.* post-training assessment 2 *vs.* post-training assessment 3) × group (DCER *vs.* control) × limb (trained *vs.* untrained) was used to analyze the 1-RM data. A two-way repeated measured ANOVA (time [training session 1 *vs.* training session 2 *vs.* training session 3] × set (1 *vs.* 2 *vs.* 3 *vs.* 4)) was used to analyze RPE assessed after each set during training. A one-way repeated measures ANOVA (time (training session 1 *vs.* training session 2 *vs.* training session 3)) was used to analyze training session RPE. When appropriate, follow-up analyses were performed using lower-order two- and one-way repeated measured ANOVAs, and paired sample *t*-tests. An alpha level of $p \leqslant 0.05$ was considered statistically significant for all comparisons. Predictive Analytics SoftWare (PASW) version 18.0.0 (SPSS Inc., Chicago, IL, USA) was used for all statistical analyses.

3. Results

3.1. Dynamic Constant External Resistance Assessments

Table 1 contains the means (±SE) for 1-RM strength in the trained and untrained leg. There was no three-way interaction for time × group × limb ($p = 0.11$). However, there was a significant two-way interaction for time × group ($p = 0.001$). Post-hoc pairwise comparisons for the marginal means indicated that 1-RM increased in both trained and untrained limbs from pre- to post-training assessment 1 for the DCER group ($p < 0.001$) (Figure 1). There were no differences in 1-RM strength for the DCER group among post-training assessments 1, 2, and 3 ($p > 0.05$) (Figure 2). No significant changes were found for the control group ($p > 0.05$).

Table 1. Means (±SE) for leg extension 1-RM.

	Group		Pre-Training Assessment 1	Post-Training Assessment 1	Post-Training Assessment 2	Post-Training Assessment 3
1-RM (kg)	DCER (*n* = 10)	Trained	43.0 ± 3.0	52.6 ± 3.8 *	50.5 ± 3.5 *	50.2 ± 3.2 *
		Untrained	41.9 ± 2.7	48.9 ± 4.2 *	48.9 ± 3.8 *	48.6 ± 3.5 *
	CONT (*n* = 9)	Trained	41.7 ± 2.2	41.9 ± 2.1	41.8 ± 1.9	42.7 ± 1.6
		Untrained	41.9 ± 2.1	41.8 ± 1.9	41.7 ± 2.0	42.2 ± 1.7

Notes: 1-RM = 1 repetition maximum; DCER = dynamic constant external resistance; CONT = control. * Denotes significant change from pre- to post-assessments.

3.2. Rating of Perceived Exertion

Table 2 contains the means (±SE) for set and session RPE from the training group. There was no two-way interaction for time × set for set RPE ($p = 0.41$). However, there was a significant main effect for set ($p < 0.001$). Post-hoc pairwise comparisons for the marginal means (collapsed across time) indicated a significant main effect for set RPE ($p < 0.05$). RPE increased significantly from the first until the last set within each session ($p < 0.05$). For session RPE, there was no main effect for time ($p = 0.55$).

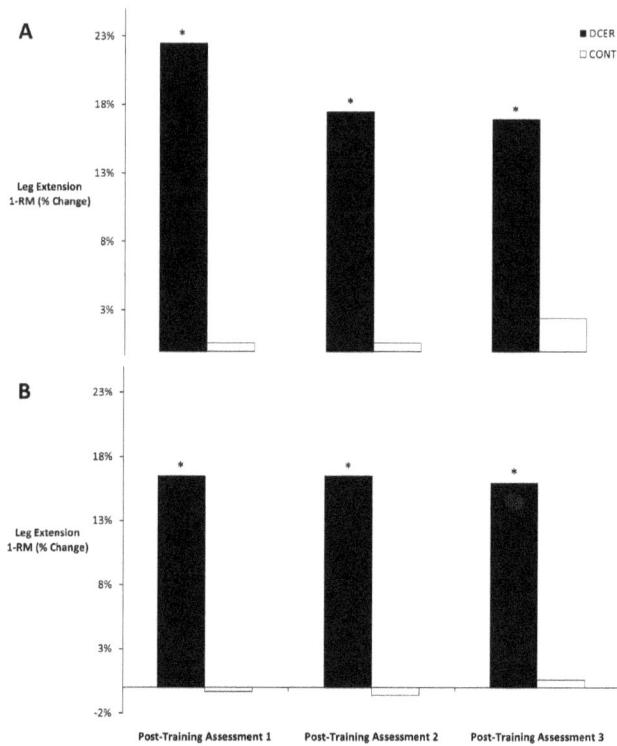

Figure 1. Means of percent change for leg extension 1-RM for the trained (**A**) and untrained (**B**) legs. * Denotes significant difference from the pre-test for the DCER group. DCER = dynamic constant external resistance; CONT = control.

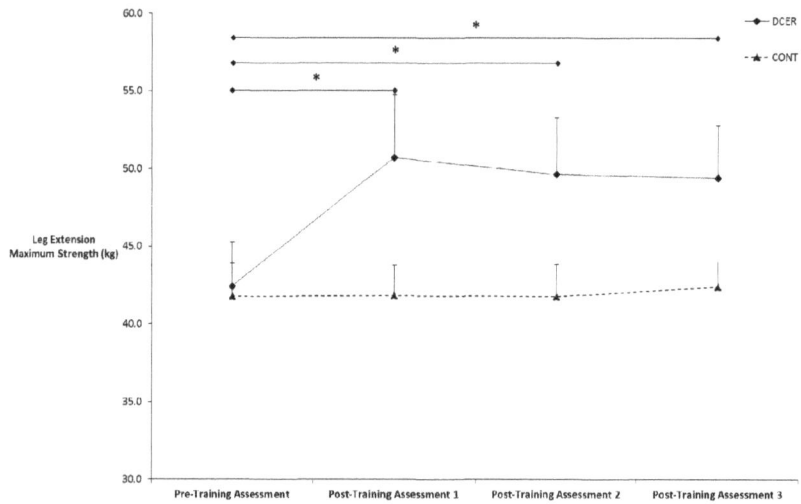

Figure 2. Means (±SE) for leg extension 1-RM collapsed across limb. * Denotes significant difference from the pre-test for the DCER group. DCER = dynamic constant external resistance; CONT = control.

Table 2. Means ($\pm$SE) for set and session rating of perceived exertion for the DCER group.

Training Session	1st Set	2nd Set	3rd Set	4th Set	Session
Session 1	6.4 ± 0.54	7.3 ± 0.63 *	8.3 ± 0.45 *	8.6 ± 0.37 *	7.6 ± 0.48
Session 2	5.4 ± 0.37	6.9 ± 0.31 *	7.8 ± 0.29 *	8.6 ± 0.43 *	7.1 ± 0.35
Session 3	5.8 ± 0.33	6.9 ± 0.43 *	7.9 ± 0.50 *	8.5 ± 0.48 *	7.5 ± 0.40

Notes: DCER = dynamic constant external resistance. * Denotes significant change over sets within each training session.

4. Discussion

Perhaps the most important finding of the present study was the increase in DCER strength acquired by the training group. DCER strength increased from pre- to post-training assessment 1 in the trained and untrained legs for the DCER training group and remained elevated during post-training assessments 2 and 3. To our knowledge, this was the first study to report DCER strength gains with short-term resistance training while also considering the detraining period of two weeks. These findings are in agreement with previous studies reporting PT increases after short-term isokinetic training [1,2]. In addition, the DCER group retained the strength gains during post-training assessments 2 and 3. That is, DCER strength remained elevated over a two-week period. Typical increases in strength obtained in longer resistance training programs are diminished after several weeks of detraining [10–14,16]. Colliander and Tesch (1992) compared the effects of resistance training and detraining using concentric-only and combined concentric and eccentric muscle actions of the leg extensors and reported that the group performing coupled concentric and eccentric muscle actions had a greater overall increase in PT after training and detraining than the concentric-only group [16]. These authors suggested strength decreases observed during detraining are not likely due to atrophy, but perhaps a reduction in neural drive or motor unit activation and hypothesized eccentric muscle actions are capable of inducing greater motor unit activation than concentric muscle actions [16]. Thus, it was suggested a resistance training program incorporating combined concentric and eccentric repetitions of leg extension can retain more of the obtained strength gains than the training program with concentric-only repetitions [16]. Likewise, Farthing (2003) found eccentric-only muscle action training elicited greater strength gains than concentric-only training [18]. Similarly, Knight *et al.*, (2001) suggested that isotonic muscle actions may be more effective at increasing torque because isokinetic resistance is accommodating, hence, it decreases with fatigue [19]. These findings [16,18,19], along with the findings of the current study may indicate an advantage of DCER over isokinetic resistance training programs when conducted over a relatively short period of time.

For the DCER training group, despite training only one leg, strength increased on the contralateral limb and was maintained over the two-week detraining period. Unilateral resistance training of a limb can increase the strength of the contralateral limb through a concept termed cross-education [27]. Increases in strength of the contralateral, untrained limb, have been extensively reported in the literature [27,28]. Possibly an important finding of the current study is that short-term resistance training also elicited the cross-education effect. This has important implications for injury rehabilitation, where in the initial period post-injury strength gains on an injured limb can conceivably be obtained with short-term contralateral resistance training. Contralateral strength gains have been hypothesized to be attributed to central neural adaptations (*i.e.*, excitation of the cortex), increased motoneuron output, and improved postural stabilization [27–29]. Accordingly, structural changes in the brain have been reported after only four weeks of unilateral resistance training concomitant with strength increases in trained and untrained limb [30]. In fact, strength gains may not be restricted to the contralateral untrained muscle, but might be observed in the contralateral untrained antagonist muscle [31]. Therefore, future studies should investigate the effects of short-term resistance training on contralateral antagonist muscles.

Strength gains were also maintained during the two-week detraining period in the DCER group. Although in the present study subjects were untrained, these findings were similar to those of Hortobagyi *et al.*, (1993), who found that two weeks of detraining of resistance-trained athletes did not cause a significant decrease in maximal bench press, squat, isometric, or concentric isokinetic strength [32]. Similarly, Shaver (1975) reported that recently acquired strength can be maintained in both trained and untrained limb for up to one week [33]. To our knowledge, the current study is the first to demonstrate short-term increases in strength can be maintained for a two-week period and in untrained limbs. In contrast, other authors have suggested strength gains that have been recently acquired may diminish faster than in strength-trained athletes [9,33]. Thus, the experience with resistance training (novice *vs.* well-trained athletes) should be considered when interpreting the results of a short-term resistance training program and its potential lasting effects.

The neuromuscular system undergoes numerous adaptations following a resistance training program [6,7,34–38]. Short-term resistance training has been shown to increase muscle strength and isokinetic performance after only a few days of training. Increases in muscular strength following a resistance training program can be attributed to neural and hypertrophic factors [6,34–37,39]. Therefore, voluntary strength increases due to not only the CSA and quality of muscle mass but also to the extent in which the muscle mass is able to activate [39]. In general, neural factors are believed to account for most of the increases in strength in the early stages of a resistance training program, whereas hypertrophic factors gradually become prevalent after several weeks of training [6,36,38–42]. Research suggests early adaptations to resistance training programs are related to improvements in neuromuscular efficiency, which perhaps indicates an increased capacity to activate skeletal muscle voluntarily [1,2,4,7,42]. Hence, initial improvements in strength and muscular performance reported following short-term resistance training are generally attributed to neural adaptations rather than muscle fiber hypertrophy [6,7]. However, the specific mechanisms of such adaptations in short-term training are not fully understood [2]. For example, Akima *et al.*, (1999) reported increases in PT after two weeks of resistance training but no changes in muscle CSA or fiber area suggesting strength increases occurred without muscle hypertrophy [7]. Similarly, Prevost *et al.*, (1999) reported velocity-specific increases in PT training at $270° \cdot s^{-1}$ after increases in PT after two days of isokinetic training but not with training at 30 and $150° \cdot s^{-1}$ [4]. Because improvements were only seen in one velocity, and muscle hypertrophy would most likely yield strength increases at the other velocities, investigators suggested that neural adaptations play a major role in strength improvements which are specific to a training velocity [4]. Beck *et al.*, (2007) suggested that responses to training might be influenced by the number of training sessions, training volume, and muscle(s) being tested [3]. Nevertheless, Akima *et al.*, (1999) and Costa *et al.*, (2013) suggested future studies should investigate the precise mechanisms underlying strength gains obtained with short-term resistance training [7,43].

The results revealed there were no differences in RPE as acknowledged by the subjects among the DCER training sessions. However, RPE increased from the first to the fourth set within each training session. These results are similar to those found by Egan *et al.*, (2006), who reported mean session RPE values of 7.3 for six sets of six repetitions of traditional resistance training using squats at an intensity of 80% of 1-RM [22]. Likewise, Sweet *et al.*, (2004) reported mean RPE values between 6.8 and 8.2 for 70 and 90% of leg press 1-RM, respectively [23]. Thus, perceived effort from a short-term resistance training program in the current study was similar to previous studies and was not lower because of the shorter training program duration.

5. Conclusions

The primary finding of this study was that DCER strength increased in the trained and untrained limbs with three days of contralateral training. This has important implications for injury rehabilitation, where in the initial period post-injury, strength gains on an injured limb can possibly be obtained with short-term resistance training. Furthermore, research has shown the feasibility and benefits of preoperative resistance training prior to surgical intervention to decrease the odds of inpatient

Sports 2016, *4*, 7

rehabilitation, reduce the length of hospital stay, and promote overall postoperative recovery [44–47]. It is believed the increases were due to an unidentified factor because of strength gains observed in the untrained limb after DCER resistance training. Future studies should investigate the precise physiological components responsible for short-term contralateral strength gains. The findings of the current study may indicate an advantage of DCER over isokinetic resistance training programs when conducted over a relatively short period of time. These findings have important implications in clinical rehabilitation settings, sports injury prevention, as well as in other allied health fields such as physical therapy, occupational therapy, and athletic training. To our knowledge, the current study is the first to demonstrate recently-acquired strength can be maintained for a two-week period in untrained limbs. Therefore, future studies should examine the effects of short-term resistance training on injury prevention and rehabilitation.

Author Contributions: Pablo B. Costa was involved in the study concept and design, and was the primary manuscript writer, and carried out data acquisition, data analysis, and data interpretation. Trent J. Herda and Ashley A. Herda were significant contributors to data acquisition, read and approved the final manuscript, and were manuscript reviewers/revisers. Joel T. Cramer was the primary manuscript reviewer/reviser, a substantial contributor to concept and design, contributed to data analysis and interpretation, and was involved in manuscript revision.

Conflicts of Interest: The authors declare no conflict of interest.

References

1. Cramer, J.T.; Stout, J.R.; Culbertson, J.Y.; Egan, A.D. Effects of creatine supplementation and three days of resistance training on muscle strength, power output, and neuromuscular function. *J. Strength Cond. Res.* **2007**, *21*, 668–677. [PubMed]
2. Coburn, J.W.; Housh, T.J.; Malek, M.H.; Weir, J.P.; Cramer, J.T.; Beck, T.W.; Johnson, G.O. Neuromuscular responses to three days of velocity-specific isokinetic training. *J. Strength Cond. Res.* **2006**, *20*, 892–898. [PubMed]
3. Beck, T.W.; Housh, T.J.; Johnson, G.O.; Weir, J.P.; Cramer, J.T.; Coburn, J.W.; Malek, M.H.; Mielke, M. Effects of two days of isokinetic training on strength and electromyographic amplitude in the agonist and antagonist muscles. *J. Strength Cond. Res.* **2007**, *21*, 757–762. [PubMed]
4. Prevost, M.C.; Nelson, A.G.; Maraj, B.K.V. The effect of two days of velocity-specific isokinetic training on torque production. *J. Strength Cond. Res.* **1999**, *13*, 35–39.
5. Brown, L.E.; Whitehurst, M. The effect of short-term isokinetic training on force and rate of velocity development. *J. Strength Cond. Res.* **2003**, *17*, 88–94. [PubMed]
6. Moritani, T.; deVries, H.A. Neural factors *versus* hypertrophy in the time course of muscle strength gain. *Am. J. Phys. Med.* **1979**, *58*, 115–130. [PubMed]
7. Akima, H.; Takahashi, H.; Kuno, S.Y.; Masuda, K.; Masuda, T.; Shimojo, H.; Anno, I.; Itai, Y.; Katsuta, S. Early phase adaptations of muscle use and strength to isokinetic training. *Med. Sci. Sports Exerc.* **1999**, *31*, 588–594. [CrossRef] [PubMed]
8. Mujika, I.; Padilla, S. Muscular characteristics of detraining in humans. *Med. Sci. Sports Exerc.* **2001**, *33*, 1297–1303. [CrossRef] [PubMed]
9. Mujika, I.; Padilla, S. Detraining: Loss of training-induced physiological and performance adaptations. Part i: Short term insufficient training stimulus. *Sports Med.* **2000**, *30*, 79–87. [CrossRef] [PubMed]
10. Hakkinen, K.; Komi, P.V.; Tesch, P.A. Effects of combined concentric and eccentric strength training and detraining on force-time, muscle fiber and metabolic characteristics of leg extensor muscles. *Scand. J. Sports Sci.* **1981**, *3*, 50–58.
11. Hakkinen, K.; Alen, M.; Komi, P.V. Changes in isometric force- and relaxation-time, electromyographic and muscle fibre characteristics of human skeletal muscle during strength training and detraining. *Acta Physiol. Scand.* **1985**, *125*, 573–585. [CrossRef] [PubMed]
12. Houston, M.E.; Froese, E.A.; Valeriote, S.P.; Green, H.J.; Ranney, D.A. Muscle performance, morphology and metabolic capacity during strength training and detraining: A one leg model. *Eur. J. Appl. Physiol. Occup. Physiol.* **1983**, *51*, 25–35. [CrossRef] [PubMed]

13. Narici, M.V.; Roi, G.S.; Landoni, L.; Minetti, A.E.; Cerretelli, P. Changes in force, cross-sectional area and neural activation during strength training and detraining of the human quadriceps. *Eur. J. Appl Physiol. Occup. Physiol.* **1989**, *59*, 310–319. [CrossRef] [PubMed]

14. Thorstensson, A. Observations on strength training and detraining. *Acta Physiol. Scand.* **1977**, *100*, 491–493. [CrossRef] [PubMed]

15. Andersen, L.L.; Andersen, J.L.; Magnusson, S.P.; Aagaard, P. Neuromuscular adaptations to detraining following resistance training in previously untrained subjects. *Eur. J. Appl. Physiol.* **2005**, *93*, 511–518. [CrossRef] [PubMed]

16. Colliander, E.B.; Tesch, P.A. Effects of detraining following short term resistance training on eccentric and concentric muscle strength. *Acta Physiol. Scand.* **1992**, *144*, 23–29. [CrossRef] [PubMed]

17. Faigenbaum, A.D.; Westcott, W.L.; Micheli, L.J.; Outerbridge, A.R.; Long, C.J.; LaRosa-Loud, R.; Zaichkowsky, L.D. The effects of strength training and detraining on children. *J. Strength Cond. Res.* **1996**, *10*, 109–114. [CrossRef]

18. Farthing, J.P.; Chilibeck, P.D. The effects of eccentric and concentric training at different velocities on muscle hypertrophy. *Eur. J. Appl Physiol.* **2003**, *89*, 578–586. [CrossRef] [PubMed]

19. Knight, K.; Ingersoll, C.; Bartholomew, J. Isotonic contractions might be more effective than isokinetic contractions in developing muscle strength. *J. Sport Rehabil.* **2001**, *10*, 124–131.

20. Weir, J.P.; Wagner, L.L.; Housh, T.J. The effect of rest interval length on repeated maximal bench presses. *J. Strength Cond. Res.* **1994**, *8*. [CrossRef]

21. Matuszak, M.E.; Fry, A.C.; Weiss, L.W.; Ireland, T.R.; McKnight, M.M. Effect of rest interval length on repeated 1 repetition maximum back squats. *J. Strength Cond. Res.* **2003**, *17*, 634–637. [PubMed]

22. Egan, A.; Winchester, J.; Foster, C.; McGuigan, M. Using session rpe to monitor different methods of resistance exercise. *J. Sports Sci. Med.* **2006**, *5*, 289–295.

23. Sweet, T.W.; Foster, C.; McGuigan, M.R.; Brice, G. Quantitation of resistance training using the session rating of perceived exertion method. *J. Strength Cond. Res.* **2004**, *18*, 796–802. [PubMed]

24. Foster, C.; Florhaug, J.A.; Franklin, J.; Gottschall, L.; Hrovatin, L.A.; Parker, S.; Doleshal, P.; Dodge, C. A new approach to monitoring exercise training. *J. Strength Cond. Res.* **2001**, *15*, 109–115. [PubMed]

25. Day, M.L.; McGuigan, M.R.; Brice, G.; Foster, C. Monitoring exercise intensity during resistance training using the session rpe scale. *J. Strength Cond. Res.* **2004**, *18*, 353–358. [PubMed]

26. Douris, P.C. The effect of isokinetic exercise on the relationship between blood lactate and muscle fatigue. *J. Orthop. Sports Phys. Ther.* **1993**, *17*, 31–35. [CrossRef] [PubMed]

27. Munn, J.; Herbert, R.D.; Gandevia, S.C. Contralateral effects of unilateral resistance training: A meta-analysis. *J. Appl. Physiol.* **2004**, *96*, 1861–1866. [CrossRef] [PubMed]

28. Carroll, T.J.; Herbert, R.D.; Munn, J.; Lee, M.; Gandevia, S.C. Contralateral effects of unilateral strength training: Evidence and possible mechanisms. *J. Appl. Physiol.* **2006**, *101*, 1514–1522. [CrossRef] [PubMed]

29. Rutherford, O.M.; Jones, D.A. The role of learning and coordination in strength training. *Eur. J. Appl. Physiol. Occup. Physiol.* **1986**, *55*, 100–105. [CrossRef] [PubMed]

30. Palmer, H.S.; Haberg, A.K.; Fimland, M.S.; Solstad, G.M.; Moe Iversen, V.; Hoff, J.; Helgerud, J.; Eikenes, L. Structural brain changes after 4 weeks of unilateral strength training of the lower limb. *J. Appl. Physiol.* **2013**, *115*, 167–175. [CrossRef] [PubMed]

31. Sariyildiz, M.; Karacan, I.; Rezvani, A.; Ergin, O.; Cidem, M. Cross-education of muscle strength: Cross-training effects are not confined to untrained contralateral homologous muscle. *Scand. J. Med. Sci. Sports* **2011**, *21*, e359–e364. [CrossRef] [PubMed]

32. Hortobagyi, T.; Houmard, J.A.; Stevenson, J.R.; Fraser, D.D.; Johns, R.A.; Israel, R.G. The effects of detraining on power athletes. *Med. Sci. Sports Exerc.* **1993**, *25*, 929–935. [PubMed]

33. Shaver, L.G. Cross transfer effects of conditioning and deconditioning on muscular strength. *Ergonomics* **1975**, *18*, 9–16. [CrossRef] [PubMed]

34. Kraemer, W.J.; Fleck, S.J.; Evans, W.J. Strength and power training: Physiological mechanisms of adaptation. *Exerc. Sport Sci. Rev.* **1996**, *24*, 363–397. [CrossRef] [PubMed]

35. Staron, R.S.; Karapondo, D.L.; Kraemer, W.J.; Fry, A.C.; Gordon, S.E.; Falkel, J.E.; Hagerman, F.C.; Hikida, R.S. Skeletal muscle adaptations during early phase of heavy-resistance training in men and women. *J. Appl. Physiol.* **1994**, *76*, 1247–1255. [PubMed]

36. Enoka, R.M. Muscle strength and its development. New perspectives. *Sports Med.* **1988**, *6*, 146–168. [CrossRef] [PubMed]
37. Sale, D.G. Influence of exercise and training on motor unit activation. *Exerc. Sport Sci. Rev.* **1987**, *15*, 95–151. [CrossRef] [PubMed]
38. Moritani, T.; deVries, H.A. Potential for gross muscle hypertrophy in older men. *J. Gerontol.* **1980**, *35*, 672–682. [CrossRef] [PubMed]
39. Sale, D.G. Neural adaptation to resistance training. *Med. Sci. Sports Exerc.* **1988**, *20*, S135–S145. [CrossRef] [PubMed]
40. Ikai, M.; Fukunaga, T. A study on training effect on strength per unit cross-sectional area of muscle by means of ultrasonic measurement. *Int. Z. Angew. Physiol.* **1970**, *28*, 173–180. [CrossRef] [PubMed]
41. Kanehisa, H.; Miyashita, M. Specificity of velocity in strength training. *Eur. J. Appl. Physiol. Occup. Physiol.* **1983**, *52*, 104–106. [CrossRef] [PubMed]
42. Knight, C.A.; Kamen, G. Adaptations in muscular activation of the knee extensor muscles with strength training in young and older adults. *J. Electromyogr. Kinesiol.* **2001**, *11*, 405–412. [CrossRef]
43. Costa, P.B.; Herda, T.J.; Walter, A.A.; Valdez, A.M.; Cramer, J.T. Effects of short-term resistance training and subsequent detraining on the electromechanical delay. *Muscle Nerve* **2013**, *48*, 135–136. [CrossRef] [PubMed]
44. Van Leeuwen, D.M.; de Ruiter, C.J.; Nolte, P.A.; de Haan, A. Preoperative strength training for elderly patients awaiting total knee arthroplasty. *Rehabil. Res. Pract.* **2014**, *2014*. [CrossRef] [PubMed]
45. Rooks, D.S.; Huang, J.; Bierbaum, B.E.; Bolus, S.A.; Rubano, J.; Connolly, C.E.; Alpert, S.; Iversen, M.D.; Katz, J.N. Effect of preoperative exercise on measures of functional status in men and women undergoing total hip and knee arthroplasty. *Arthritis Rheum.* **2006**, *55*, 700–708. [CrossRef] [PubMed]
46. Topp, R.; Swank, A.M.; Quesada, P.M.; Nyland, J.; Malkani, A. The effect of prehabilitation exercise on strength and functioning after total knee arthroplasty. *PM R* **2009**, *1*, 729–735. [CrossRef] [PubMed]
47. Swank, A.M.; Kachelman, J.B.; Bibeau, W.; Quesada, P.M.; Nyland, J.; Malkani, A.; Topp, R.V. Prehabilitation before total knee arthroplasty increases strength and function in older adults with severe osteoarthritis. *J. Strength Cond. Res.* **2011**, *25*, 318–325. [CrossRef] [PubMed]

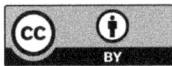

![sports]

sports

MDPI

Article

Effects of Respiratory Muscle Warm-up on High-Intensity Exercise Performance

Taylor S. Thurston, Jared W. Coburn, Lee E. Brown, Albert Bartolini, Tori L. Beaudette, Patrick Karg, Kathryn A. McLeland, Jose A. Arevalo, Daniel A. Judelson and Andrew J. Galpin *

Center for Sport Performance, Department of Kinesiology, California State University, Fullerton, CA 92834, USA; taylor.thurston@utah.edu (T.S.T.); Jcoburn@fullerton.edu (J.W.C.); leebrown@fullerton.edu (L.E.B.); abartolini@fullerton.edu (A.B.); TBeaudette@csusb.edu (T.L.B.); pkarg@fullerton.edu (P.K.); k.a.mcleland@gmail.com (K.A.M.); jarevalo@fullerton.edu (J.A.A.); dan.judelson@nike.com (D.A.J.)

* Correspondence: agalpin@fullerton.edu; Tel.: +1-657-278-2112; Fax: +1-657-278-5317

Academic Editor: Eling de Bruin

Received: 21 September 2015; Accepted: 30 October 2015; Published: 5 November 2015

Abstract: Exercise performance is partially limited by the functionality of the respiratory musculature. Training these muscles improves steady-state exercise performance. However, less is known about the efficacy of executing a respiratory muscle warm-up (RWU) immediately prior to high-intensity exercise. Our study purpose was to use a practitioner-friendly airflow restriction device to investigate the effects of a high, medium, or low intensity RWU on short, high-intensity exercise and pulmonary, cardiovascular, and metabolic function. Eleven recreationally active, males (24.9 ± 4.2 y, 178.8 ± 9.0 cm, 78.5 ± 10.4 kg, 13.4% ± 4.2% body fat) cycled at 85% peak power to exhaustion (TTE) following four different RWU conditions (separate days, in random order): (1) high; (2) medium; (3) low airflow inspiration restriction, or no RWU. When analyzed as a group, TTE did not improve following any RWU (4.73 ± 0.33 min). However, 10 of the 11 participants improved ≥25 s in one of the three RWU conditions (average = 47.6 ± 13.2 s), which was significantly better than ($p < 0.05$) the control trial (CON). Neither blood lactate nor perceived difficulty was altered by condition. In general, respiratory exchange ratios were significantly lower during the early stages of TTE in all RWU conditions. Our findings suggest RWU efficacy is predicated on identifying optimal inspiration intensity, which clearly differs between individuals.

Keywords: intervals; high-intensity; performance; respiratory; hypoxia; breathing; restriction; hypocapnia; fatigue

---

1. Introduction

Numerous physiological factors such as pH, temperature, neurological input, and substrate availability limit exercise performance. One particularly understudied aspect is the role of the respiratory musculature. The available literature provides clear evidence that fatigue of this system hampers exercise performance [1–4] by inducing a metaboreflex response, which causes sympathetic outflow and a resulting vasoconstriction/reduced oxygen delivery to working muscles [3,5–9]. Fortunately, functional capacity of the respiratory musculature is modifiable. Intentionally restricting airflow during inhalation, exhalation, or both [10–12] forces the respiratory muscles to increase work output to adequately support airflow and gas exchange needs. Improvements in whole-body performance have been found in a variety of sports [12–15] and general exercise settings [16–18] following these types of respiratory exercise. For example, Romer, McConnell, and Jones (2002) reported that chronic respiratory training significantly improved 20 km and 40 km cycling time trial performance by ~3%–5% [12].

Restrictive airflow breathing activities may also improve acute exercise performance by functioning as a pre-exercise respiratory muscle warm-up (RWU). This is of particular importance when engaging in high-intensity exercise. The respiratory muscles have high aerobic capacities, multiple sources of blood supply, and a unique resilience to vasoconstriction; making them naturally fatigue-resistant to low-moderate exercise intensities. However, they are susceptible to fatigue when exercising at intensities greater than 80% of VO_2max for prolonged periods of time [5]. Volianitis and colleagues (1999) understood this phenomenon and sought to examine whether or not a RWU (which presumably improves function of the respiratory muscles) could sufficiently alter high intensity exercise performance.

This was accomplished by comparing performance during a six-minute maximal rowing test following either a sport-specific warm-up or a RWU. The researchers noted the RWU induced a significant increase in rowing distance of 18 m. On the contrary, Johnson *et al.*, (2014) found no change in 10 km cycling time trial performance following a RWU combined with a sport specific warm-up (compared to a sport specific warm-up alone). Thus, while RWU appears helpful when utilized prior to short duration, high-intensity rowing, its effectiveness may be eliminated when cycling. Further examination of this speculation is important given the popularity of high-intensity cycling among personal trainers, strength and conditioning coaches, and health professionals.

Confusing the matter even more, the intensity (*i.e.*, amount of airflow restriction) and volume of the RWU significantly affect its outcome. Most studies report success when implementing two sets of 30 respiratory cycles at 40% of maximal inspiratory pressure [1–15,18]. Higher intensity restriction actually fatigues the system, while less restriction is insufficient [19]. Measurement of maximal inspiratory pressure typically requires specialized, expensive equipment. Practitioners attempting to implement a RWU are unlikely to possess such devices. However, less expensive RWU devices that allow manipulation of airflow restriction intensity are commercially available, but lack scientific scrutiny. Therefore, the purpose of this study was to utilize one of these practitioner friendly devices to investigate the effects of a high, medium, or low intensity RWU on cycling time to exhaustion and pulmonary, cardiovascular, and metabolic function.

2. Materials and Method

2.1. Study Design

This study was designed to investigate the effectiveness of three different RWU intensities on exercise performance. Day 1 consisted of baseline measurements and familiarization of the RWU protocol. On Days 2–5, participants performed a RWU with either high (HI), medium (MID), or low (LO) amounts of airflow restriction (or no RWU CON) immediately prior to a cycling test to exhaustion (TTE). Each trial (HI, MID, LO, CON) was separated by at least 48 h, and the order of each trial was randomized. Exercise performance and measures of pulmonary, cardiovascular, and metabolic function were collected and analyzed during each of the four trials.

2.2. Study Controls

Trial order was randomized via a Latin Squares design, with each trial occurring at least 48, but no more than 96, h apart. All trials occurred in the morning between 6:00 and 10:00 am, with each trial occurring ±1 h from the first experimental visit for each individual participant. To ensure training status did not change throughout the study, participants kept a training log for the week prior to their first testing session. Activity levels were then mimicked and recorded their throughout the duration of their involvement in the study. Participants were asked to refrain from exercise for the 36 h before testing and were encouraged to sleep ≥8 h the night before each test. Similar measures were taken for dietary intake during the 24 h period that preceded each individual testing session. Participants fasted 12 h prior to each testing session. Nonetheless, three participants were removed from the study because of significant differences in their carbohydrate intake the 24 h prior to one or more of their trials. To ensure sufficient hydration, participants were instructed to drink water the night before (~1000 mL) and the morning of (~500 mL) testing. Hydration status was monitored via urine specific gravity analysis prior to each trial. Recordings of greater than 1.020 resulted in a rescheduling of the exercise trial [20]. No external motivation (e.g., cheering, yelling, music, *etc.*) was provided or allowed during the RWU, pulmonary testing, or the TTE.

2.3. Participants

Fourteen healthy male recreational exercisers enrolled in the study, but three were removed from the final analyses (*n* = 11, Table 1). Participants were excluded prior to beginning any activities of the study if they had any prior experience with RWU (or similar) practices. Inclusion criteria required participants be free from any cardiovascular, metabolic, and pulmonary diseases or illnesses that may affect the pulmonary system, or have any joint, musculoskeletal, and/or neuromuscular injuries or pain that may affect their ability to perform maximal cycling exercise. To ensure adequate levels of aerobic fitness, participants were also required to demonstrate a VO_2max of ≥45 mL·kg^1·min^{-1}. Prior to participating, all volunteers were informed of the risks and signed a document of informed consent. This document, as well as the study, were approved by The University Institutional Review Board.

Table 1. Participant descriptive information.

Variable	Mean ± SD
Age (y)	24.9 ± 4.2
Height (cm)	178.8 ± 9.0
Mass (kg)	78.5 ± 10.4
Body Fat (%)	13.4 ± 4.2
VO_{2max} (mL·kg^{-1}·min^{-1})	54.8 ± 6.9
Cycling Intensity (W)	274.5 ± 45.8

2.4. Preliminary Testing

During Visit 1, investigators assessed height and mass via stadiometer (SECA, Ontario, CA, USA) and an electronic scale (Healthometer Toledo ES200L, Ohaus, Pine Brook, NJ, USA), respectively. Body fat percentage was calculated via a three site skinfold protocol from the chest, thigh, and abdomen [21]. Participants then performed a cycle ergometer (Ergomedic 839E, Monarch, Stockholm, Sweden) VO_2max test. Expired gasses were measured using a TRUEMAX 2400 metabolic cart (PARVOMEDICS, Sandy, UT, USA), calibrated before each trial. The test required participants to initially cycle at 50 W for five minutes. The test subsequently increased 25 W every minute until the participant was too exhausted to continue, VO_2 plateaued, heart rate (HR) (Polar Electro Inc., FS1 and TS1, Woodbury, NY, USA) failed to increase despite increasing intensity, a respiratory exchange ratio (RER) greater than 1.15 was achieved, or the participant indicated a rating of perceived exertion (RPE) of greater than 18 [22]. Following the VO_2max test, participants were familiarized with the RWU protocol. This consisted of 2 sets of 30 breaths (1 min rest between sets) [19] while the nose was clipped shut and an air flow inhalation restriction device (O_2 Trainer™, Westwood, CA, USA) was placed in the mouth. The device (Figure 1) was set to the highest restriction setting possible during the familiarization for all participants to ensure they were capable of completing the protocol during HI. Participants were instructed to both inhale and exhale with maximum effort per breath.

2.5. Experimental Trials

Visit 2–5 consisted of either a RWU with HI, MID, or LO airflow restriction, or no RWU of any type (CON), followed by TTE. RWU was accomplished by performing 2 sets of 30 repetitions (1 min rest between sets) of maximal breaths at their normal breathing cadence. During CON, participants rested quietly on the cycle and performed no respiratory warm-up. The time between the end of the warm-up and the start of TTE was matched between all four experimental conditions. Participants used the same device for all familiarization and experimental trials. The specific RWU volumes and intra-set rest intervals used here replicated procedure used in previous studies [13–18]. The device was specifically chosen because it is inexpensive, portable, and allows the amount of airflow restriction to be adjusted (range of 3–13 mm), making it a realistic option for practitioners. Moreover, the device includes a three way valve built into the mouthpiece allowing airflow to be restricted during inhalation, yet unrestricted during exhalation. To contribute to this literature regarding optimal inspiratory intensity, we included RWU conditions across the spectrum of airflow inhalation restriction allowed by the device. Linear changes in airflow restriction diameter settings on the device likely translate into exponential changes in flow rate and/or inspiratory pressure. Thus, we chose to perform HI with a 3 mm opening (fitting #13), MID with an 8 mm opening (fitting #7), and LO with a 13 mm opening (fitting #2).

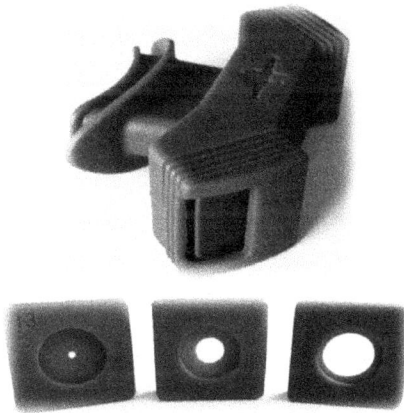

Figure 1. Photo of airflow restriction device used for the respiratory warm-up. Interchangeable caps are placed on one side of the device, restricting inhalation of air to the desired diameter, but allowing unrestricted exhalation. The high restriction (HI) warm-up used the 3 mm opening (fitting #13), the medium restriction (MID) used the 8 mm opening (fitting #7), and the low restriction (LO) used the 13 mm opening (fitting #2).

Upon arrival at the laboratory for all experimental trials, participants were assessed for hydration and training/nutrition logs were examined. After verifying compliance with all pre-study controls, participants were fitted to the cycle ergometer and the metabolic mask was sized to the participant's head and mouth. Personal cycle settings were recorded and reproduced for subsequent trials. After a five minute rest, blood lactate was measured via finger prick of the index finger (Accutrend Lactate Analyzer, Roche Diagnostics, Basel, Switzerland). Participants then performed pulmonary function testing via spirometry (SpiroLab II, SDI Diagnostics, Easton, MA, USA) until three repeatable values were recorded.

Volunteers then performed a five minute warm-up at 50 W on the cycle ergometer. Then, while remaining on the cycle, they performed the appropriate RWU protocol. Another pulmonary function assessment was conducted following the completion of the last set of RWU. This testing, and all pre-TTE preparations (e.g., mask set-up, *etc.*) were completed within two minutes of completing the cycling warm-up. TTE was performed at 85% of the participants adjusted peak wattage (achieved during the VO$_2$max test). RPE was measured at 1 min intervals using the Borg 6–20 scale. Volume of oxygen exhaled (VO$_2$), volume of carbon dioxide exhaled (VCO$_2$), RER, minute ventilation (VE), and HR were recorded using 15 s averages during the TTE. The TTE was terminated when the exerciser failed to maintain $\geq$60 revolutions per minute for five consecutive seconds [23,24]. Blood lactate was taken immediately after TTE was terminated. Five minutes of rest on the ergometer was given to participants before a post-exercise pulmonary function test was completed.

2.6. Statistical Analyses

Performance during TTE was analyzed by using a 4 (RWU Intensity) × 1 (time) repeated measures analysis of variance (ANOVA). A 4 (RWU Intensity) × 2 (pre and post TTE) repeated ANOVA was used to assess statistical differences among treatments for blood lactate. A 4 (RWU Intensity) × 6 (pre, 1 min, 2 min, 3 min, 4 min, and post TTE) repeated ANOVA was used to assess statistical differences among treatments for RPE. A *t*-test was used to compare the each individual's best performance against CON. Forced vital capacity (FVC), forced expiratory volume in 1 s (FEV_1), forced expiratory volume percentage (FEV1%), forced inspiratory vital capacity (FIVC), and peak expiratory flow (PEF) were analyzed via separate 4 (RWU Intensity) × 3 (baseline, post RWU/pre TTE, and post TTE) repeated ANOVA. Metabolic data were analyzed only to the point of the earliest TTE. Thus, 4 (RWU Intensity) × 13 (time) repeated ANOVA were used to assess statistical differences among treatments for absolute VO_2, VCO_2, RER, VE, and HR. In the presence of a significant F ratio, Tukey's post hoc test was used to analyze pair-wise comparisons. The alpha level was set at 0.05.

3. Results

3.1. Time to Exhaustion

There were no significant differences ($p \geq 0.05$) across conditions for TTE (4.73 ± 0.33 min). However, 10 of the 11 participants displayed a noticeable improvement ($\geq$25 s) in one of the three experimental conditions (HI, MID, or LO) when compared to CON. Five had their best performance during MID (Figure 2), three during LO (Figure 3), and two during HI (Figure 4). The average improvement among these best trials was 47.6 ± 13.2 s, which was significantly different than CON.

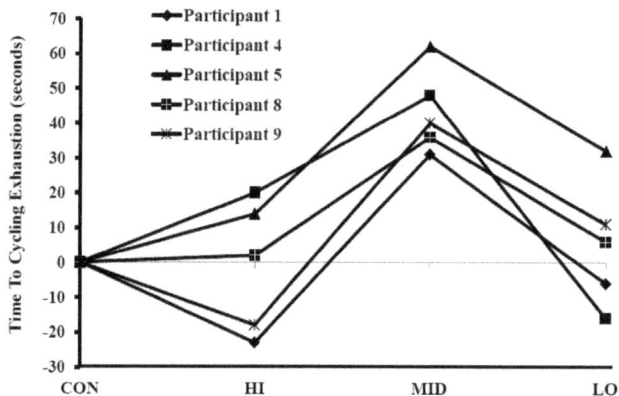

Figure 2. Changes in time to exhaustion during a cycling test immediately following a respiratory warm-up, which consisted of two sets of 30 repeitions of maximal breathes while wearing an air flow inhalation restriction device set at 13 mm (HI), 8 mm (MID), or 3 mm (LO) of restriction. A control trial (CON) was performed with no warm-up. Performance during CON was considered zero. The amount of time (seconds) more or less than CON is plotted above for each participant who experienced their best perfomrance during MID.

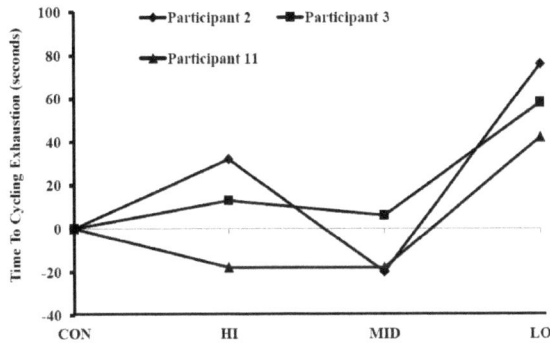

Figure 3. Changes in time to exhaustion during a cycling test immediately following a respiratory warm-up, which consisted of two sets of 30 repeitions of maximal breathes while wearing an air flow inhalation restriction device set at 13 mm (HI), 8 mm (MID), or 3 mm (LO) of restriction. A control trial (CON) was performed with no warm-up. Performance during CON was considered zero. The amount of time (seconds) more or less than CON is plotted above for each participant who experienced their best perfomrance during LO.

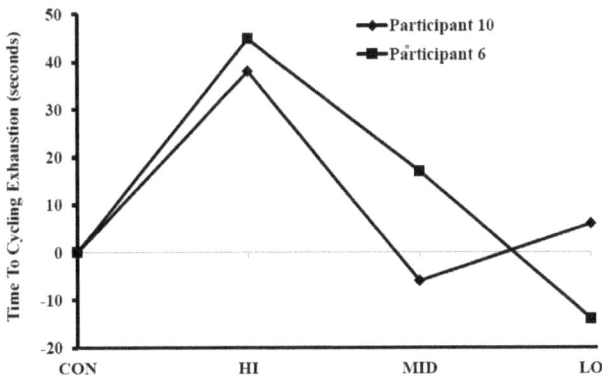

Figure 4. Changes in time to exhaustion during a cycling test immediately following a respiratory warm-up, which consisted of two sets of 30 repeitions of maximal breathes while wearing an air flow inhalation restriction device set at 3 mm (LO), 8 mm (MID, or 13 mm (HI) of restriction. A control trial (CON) was performed with no warm-up. Performance during CON was considered zero. The amount of time (seconds) more or less than CON is plotted above for each participant who experienced their best perfomrance during HI.

3.2. Rating of Perceived Exertion and Lactate

There were significant main effects, but not condition interactions, of time for lactate (Table 2) or RPE (Pre = 7.8 ± 1.4, Post = 20.0 ± 0.0).

Table 2. Lactate before and after a time to exhaustion trial. Data are reported as mean ± SD.

Condition	Pre	Post
HI	1.95 ± 0.56	15.38 ± 4.49
MID	1.91 ± 0.40	15.80 ± 4.03
LOW	2.17 ± 0.82	13.74 ± 4.14
CON	1.88 ± 0.47	14.20 ± 3.70

3.3. Pulmonary Function

No time main effects, condition main effects, or time by condition interactions were reported for FVC, FEV_1, $FEV_1\%$, or FIVC. A significant main effect of time and an interaction by condition existed for PEF. Baseline (10.33 ± 1.54, 10.33 ± 1.48, 10.33 ± 1.49 L/s) and post TTE (10.26 ± 1.47, 10.36 ± 1.70, 10.35 ± 1.61) were not different from each other, but were both significantly greater than post RWU (9.89 ± 1.55, 9.88 ± 1.84, 9.68 ± 1.42) for HI, MID, and CON, respectively. Baseline PEF (10.30 ± 1.68) was significantly greater than both post RWU (9.80 ± 1.81) and post TTE (10.06 ± 1.80) during LO.

3.4. Gas Exchange

A main effect of time was statistically significant for VCO_2, VO_2, RER, and HR. However, interaction effects between condition and time were only significant for VCO_2, RER, and VE, while a trend ($p < 0.10$) existed for VO_2. Regarding VCO2, CON was significantly greater than MID for all time points up to one minute and 30 s. For time points between 45 s and one minute and 30 s, CON was significantly greater than LOW. Regarding RER, CON was significantly higher than HI, MID, and LO for all time points up to one minute and 30 s, and higher than MID for all time points up to two minutes and 30 s. For VE, CON was significantly greater than LOW and MID, and HI was significantly greater than MID at the one-minute time point.

4. Discussion

The primary findings of this study indicate the effectiveness of the inspiratory RWU is highly contingent upon the intensity (*i.e.*, amount of airflow restriction) being optimized for the individual. If accomplished, the RWU protocol resulted in statistically significant and practically important changes in short-term, cycling to exhaustion performance. Our results also suggest that RWU, regardless of intensity, significantly decreased early stage (of exercise) RER, without altering blood lactate or perceived exertion, or decreasing exercise performance.

4.1. Performance

The interpretation that our RWU provided no performance benefit also holds merit as all conditions (HI, MID, and LO) failed to reach statistical significance. Several potential explanations exist. Firstly, the time between our RWU and the start of our exercise differed from some of the previous research. The current study followed the general methods of previous literature with similar procedures [16,18]. However, we chose to implement a rest interval that was shorter than previous research as it better reflected practices during normal exercise settings. Others have found performance enhancements when engaging in the RWU 30 min before exercise [25,26]. The optimal rest interval between RWU and exercise remains unclear, but our findings, combined with previous research [25,26], suggest longer may be better than shorter. Secondly, the limitations of the RWU device precluded us from controlling and/or quantifying inspiratory pressure or flow rate during the RWU, meaning we could not standardize conditions between or within participants. This directly influenced our grouped performance results.

Most previous research in this area has focused on identifying physiological mechanisms associated with RWU, not necessarily practitioner-friendly applications. This important stage in the research required scientists to control and monitor as many variables as possible [13–18], and led to the prescription of a desired inspiratory pressure of 40% [19]. Our goal was to examine RWU in setting more realistic to practitioners. Thus, we chose to use an inexpensive, commercially available device, knowing it could not be set to an optimal airflow restriction (per participant) *a priori*. We directly examined the loading intensity issue by asking participants to repeat the TTE trial under three different settings (which spanned the ability of the device, and was reasonable to complete the protocol). Finding significant differences among conditions was therefore difficult because of the high deviations in performance between each person's trials. This was particularly evident by the participants who had decreases in performance of ≥ 18 s (when compared to CON) during HI. These findings support previous research and suggest an optimal range exists for the intensity of a RWU, with too low of an intensity failing to produce benefit and too high of an intensity causing premature respiratory muscle fatigue [19]. However, significant improvements ($p < 0.05$) in performance were noted when the best trial per person was compared to their own CON trial. No clear patterns emerged among participants who performed best at a given RWU intensity. In conclusion: (1) an ideal inspiratory pressure exists; (2) previous research shows significant benefits of respiratory training [13,14,17,18]; and (3) individualized performance benefits of 10 of the 11 participants were more than double the standard deviation (± 20 s) better than CON during at least one of the RWU conditions. This collective evidence allows us the confidence to conclude the protocol has the potential to provide practically important benefits to the physical performance test. The viability of a RWU under different circumstances deserves further investigation. For example, our RWU protocol only targeted the inspiratory muscles. Protocols which target the expiratory muscles (or both) may yield different findings.

4.2. Metabolic Function

The RWU significantly altered ventilation and O_2/CO_2, at least during the first two minutes of exercise. Specifically, the decrease in RER appeared to mirror those of VCO_2, but over a slightly longer time point. This was matched by a corresponding increase in VO_2 (trend). These factors could explain the enhanced VE displayed during the first minute of exercise, and combine to suggest the RWU induced arterial hypocapnia. Unfortunately, this speculation cannot be confirmed as measurement of endtidal CO_2 during the RWU was not possible. Previous studies have found hyperventilation-induced hypocapnia increases locomotor vasoconstriction, decreases muscle perfusion, and reduces O_2 delivery [27,28], which should combine to produce a diminution of exercise performance. Yet, here we report performance enhancement. Explanation of this apparent conundrum is not directly possible with the given data as specific examination of the interplay between RWU and hypocapnia requires an entirely different study design and focus. The authors can only speculate that either hypocapnia did not occur, or the RWU offset any potential detriments.

4.3. Blood Lactate and Pulmonary Function

Blood lactate was not different between RWU conditions, meaning it does not explain the changes in performance. Similar conclusions were reported in other related studies [14–16]. As expected, performance enhancements cannot be explained by acute changes in pulmonary function either as it was also generally unresponsive to the RWU, which was expected [4,12,14,29–31]. PEF did show condition specific responses, but the magnitude of change (<8%) indicates a limited clinical relevance [32]. Researchers should consider designing future research in a manner that allows specific evaluation of the pulmonary, metabolic, perceptual, muscular, neurological or other mechanisms responsible for performance enhancements.

5. Conclusions

The current study provides unique insight into the effects of RWU. Our data indicate RWU may enhance short-term, high-intensity exercise performance, but only when performed at an optimal intensity (*i.e.*, airflow restriction). Practitioners should implement with caution as intensity differs between individuals, and too difficult of a RWU hinders exercise performance. Further examination of the relationship between (1) performance-based classifications of optimal airflow restriction and (2) previously established guidelines of 40% maximum inspiratory pressure [19] would provide validation to both approaches and afford coaches/users the ability to effectively incorporate RWU into practice. It is unknown if other warm-up protocols (e.g., different volumes, longer rest between RWU, *etc.*) provide similar benefits. Moreover, the effectiveness of this RWU on exercise of other intensities, durations, or modes (e.g., running, rowing, swimming, *etc.*) is unknown. Researchers should also apply a similar, application-based research approach to study participants from other populations, particularly those with cardiopulmonary abnormalities. Further investigations in this area would benefit both the scientific community and practitioners.

Acknowledgments: The research team would like to thank all the participants for their hard work and effort in this exhausting task.

Author Contributions: Taylor S. Thurston, Jared W. Coburn, Lee E. Brown, Daniel A. Judelson and Andrew J. Galpin conceived and designed the experiments; Taylor S. Thurston, Albert Bartolini, Tori L. Beaudette, Patrick Karg, Kathryn A. McLeland, and Jose A. Arevalo performed the experiments; Taylor S. Thurston, Jared W. Coburn, Lee E. Brown, Daniel A. Judelson, and Andrew J. Galpin analyzed the data; Andrew J. Galpin contributed reagents/materials/analysis tools; Taylor S. Thurston, Jared W. Coburn, Lee E. Brown, Daniel A. Judelson and Andrew J. Galpin wrote the paper.

Conflicts of Interest: The authors declare no conflict of interest.

References

1. Mador, M.J.; Acevedo, F.A. Effect of respiratory muscle fatigue on subsequent exercise performance. *J. Appl. Physiol.* **1991**, *70*, 2059–2065. [PubMed]
2. Verges, S.; Sager, Y.; Erni, C.; Spengler, C.M. Expiratory muscle fatigue impairs exercise performance. *Eur. J. Appl. Physiol.* **2007**, *101*, 225–232. [CrossRef] [PubMed]
3. Romer, L.M.; Polkey, M.I. Exercise-induced respiratory muscle fatigue: Implications for performance. *J. Appl. Physiol.* **2008**, *104*, 879–888. [CrossRef] [PubMed]
4. Volianitis, S.; McConnell, A.K.; Jones, D.A. Assessment of maximum inspiratory pressure. Prior submaximal respiratory muscle activity ("warm-up") enhances maximum inspiratory activity and attenuates the learning effect of repeated measurement. *Respir. Int. Rev. Thorac. Dis.* **2001**, *68*, 22–27.
5. Dempsey, J.A.; Romer, L.; Rodman, J.; Miller, J.; Smith, C. Consequences of exercise-induced respiratory muscle work. *Respir. Physiol. Neurobiol.* **2006**, *151*, 242–250. [CrossRef] [PubMed]
6. Hill, J.M. Discharge of group iv phrenic afferent fibers increases during diaphragmatic fatigue. *Brain Res.* **2000**, *856*, 240–244. [CrossRef]
7. Jammes, Y.; Balzamo, E. Changes in afferent and efferent phrenic activities with electrically induced diaphragmatic fatigue. *J. Appl. Physiol.* **1992**, *73*, 894–902. [PubMed]
8. Harms, C.A.; Babcock, M.A.; McClaran, S.R.; Pegelow, D.F.; Nickele, G.A.; Nelson, W.B.; Dempsey, J.A. Respiratory muscle work compromises leg blood flow during maximal exercise. *J. Appl. Physiol.* **1997**, *82*, 1573–1583. [PubMed]
9. Sheel, A.W.; Derchak, P.A.; Morgan, B.J.; Pegelow, D.F.; Jacques, A.J.; Dempsey, J.A. Fatiguing inspiratory muscle work causes reflex reduction in resting leg blood flow in humans. *J. Physiol.* **2001**, *537*, 277–289. [CrossRef] [PubMed]
10. Verges, S.; Lenherr, O.; Haner, A.C.; Schulz, C.; Spengler, C.M. Increased fatigue resistance of respiratory muscles during exercise after respiratory muscle endurance training. *Am. J. Physiol. Regul. Integr. Comp. Physiol.* **2007**, *292*, R1246–R1253. [CrossRef] [PubMed]
11. Verges, S.; Renggli, A.S.; Notter, D.A.; Spengler, C.M. Effects of different respiratory muscle training regimes on fatigue-related variables during volitional hyperpnoea. *Respir. Physiol. Neurobiol.* **2009**, *169*, 282–290. [CrossRef] [PubMed]
12. Romer, L.M.; McConnell, A.K.; Jones, D.A. Inspiratory muscle fatigue in trained cyclists: Effects of inspiratory muscle training. *Med. Sci. Sports Exerc.* **2002**, *34*, 785–792. [CrossRef] [PubMed]
13. Volianitis, S.; McConnell, A.K.; Koutedakis, Y.; Jones, D.A. Specific respiratory warm-up improves rowing performance and exertional dyspnea. *Med. Sci. Sports Exerc.* **2001**, *33*, 1189–1193. [CrossRef] [PubMed]
14. Wilson, E.E.; McKeever, T.M.; Lobb, C.; Sherriff, T.; Gupta, L.; Hearson, G.; Martin, N.; Lindley, M.R.; Shaw, D.E. Respiratory muscle specific warm-up and elite swimming performance. *Br. J. Sports Med.* **2013**, *48*, 789–791. [CrossRef] [PubMed]
15. Lin, H.; Tong, T.K.; Huang, C.; Nie, J.; Lu, K.; Quach, B. Specific inspiratory muscle warm-up enhances badminton footwork performance. *Appl. Physiol. Nutr. Metab. Physiol. Appl. Nutr. Metab.* **2007**, *32*, 1082–1088. [CrossRef] [PubMed]

16. Cheng, C.F.; Tong, T.K.; Kuo, Y.C.; Chen, P.H.; Huang, H.W.; Lee, C.L. Inspiratory muscle warm-up attenuates muscle deoxygenation during cycling exercise in women athletes. *Respir. Physiol. Neurobiol.* **2013**, *186*, 296–302. [CrossRef] [PubMed]

17. Tong, T.K.; Fu, F.H. Effect of specific inspiratory muscle warm-up on intense intermittent run to exhaustion. *Eur. J. Appl. Physiol.* **2006**, *97*, 673–680. [CrossRef] [PubMed]

18. Lomax, M.; Grant, I.; Corbett, J. Inspiratory muscle warm-up and inspiratory muscle training: Separate and combined effects on intermittent running to exhaustion. *J. Sports Sci.* **2011**, *29*, 563–569. [CrossRef] [PubMed]

19. Roussos, C.S.; Macklem, P.T. Diaphragmatic fatigue in man. *J. Appl. Physiol. Respir. Environ. Exerc. Physiol.* **1977**, *43*, 189–197. [PubMed]

20. Armstrong, L.E.; Maresh, C.M.; Castellani, J.W.; Bergeron, M.F.; Kenefick, R.W.; LaGasse, K.E.; Riebe, D. Urinary indices of hydration status. *Int. J. Sport Nutr.* **1994**, *4*, 265–279. [PubMed]

21. Jackson, A.S.; Pollock, M.L. Practical assessment of body composition. *Phys. Sports Med.* **1985**, *13*, 76–90.

22. American College of Sports Medicine. *Acsm's Guidelines for Exercise Testing and Prescription*, 7th ed.; Lippincott Williams & Wilkins: Philadelphia, PA, USA, 2006; p. 366.

23. Ghosh, A.K.; Rahaman, A.A.; Singh, R. Combination of sago and soy-protein supplementation during endurance cycling exercise and subsequent high-intensity endurance capacity. *Int. J. Sport Nutr. Exerc. Metab.* **2010**, *20*, 216–223. [PubMed]

24. Ferguson-Stegall, L.; McCleave, E.L.; Ding, Z.; Kammer, L.M.; Wang, B.; Doerner, P.G.; Liu, Y.; Ivy, J.L. The effect of a low carbohydrate beverage with added protein on cycling endurance performance in trained athletes. *J. Strength Cond. Res.* **2010**, *24*, 2577–2586. [CrossRef] [PubMed]

25. Volianitis, S.; McConnell, A.K.; Koutedakis, Y.; Jones, D.A. The influence of prior activity upon inspiratory muscle strength in rowers and non-rowers. *Int. J. Sports Med.* **1999**, *20*, 542–547. [CrossRef] [PubMed]

26. Johnson, M.A.; Gregson, I.R.; Mills, D.E.; Gonzalez, J.T.; Sharpe, G.R. Inspiratory muscle warm-up does not improve cycling time-trial performance. *Eur. J. Appl. Physiol.* **2014**, *114*, 1821–1830. [CrossRef] [PubMed]

27. Chin, L.M.; Heigenhauser, G.J.; Paterson, D.H.; Kowalchuk, J.M. Effect of voluntary hyperventilation with supplemental CO_2 on pulmonary O_2 uptake and leg blood flow kinetics during moderate-intensity exercise. *Exp. Physiol.* **2013**, *98*, 1668–1682. [CrossRef] [PubMed]

28. Fan, J.L.; Bourdillon, N.; Kayser, B. Effect of end-tidal CO_2 clamping on cerebrovascular function, oxygenation, and performance during 15-km time trial cycling in severe normobaric hypoxia: The role of cerebral O_2 delivery. *Physiol. Rep.* **2013**, *1*. [CrossRef] [PubMed]

29. Enright, S.J.; Unnithan, V.B.; Heward, C.; Withnall, L.; Davies, D.H. Effect of high-intensity inspiratory muscle training on lung volumes, diaphragm thickness, and exercise capacity in subjects who are healthy. *Phys. Ther.* **2006**, *86*, 345–354. [PubMed]

30. Kilding, A.E.; Brown, S.; McConnell, A.K. Inspiratory muscle training improves 100 and 200 m swimming performance. *Eur. J. Appl. Physiol.* **2010**, *108*, 505–511. [CrossRef] [PubMed]

31. Romer, L.M.; McConnell, A.K. Specificity and reversibility of inspiratory muscle training. *Med. Sci. Sports Exerc.* **2003**, *35*, 237–244. [CrossRef] [PubMed]

32. Jain, P.; Kavuru, M.S. A practical guide for peak expiratory flow monitoring in asthma patients. *Clevel. Clin. J. Med.* **1997**, *64*, 195–202. [CrossRef]

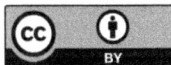

sports

MDPI

Article

Individual Responses for Muscle Activation, Repetitions, and Volume during Three Sets to Failure of High- (80% 1RM) *versus* Low-Load (30% 1RM) Forearm Flexion Resistance Exercise

Nathaniel D. M. Jenkins [1,*], **Terry J. Housh** [1], **Samuel L. Buckner** [2], **Haley C. Bergstrom** [3], **Kristen C. Cochrane** [1], **Cory M. Smith** [1], **Ethan C. Hill** [1], **Richard J. Schmidt** [1] **and Joel T. Cramer** [1,*]

[1] Department of Nutrition and Health Sciences, 211 Ruth Leverton Hall, University of Nebraska-Lincoln, Lincoln, NE 68583, USA; thoush1@unl.edu (T.J.H.); kcochrane@unl.edu (K.C.C.); csmith@unl.edu (C.M.S.); ethan.hill@unl.edu (E.C.H.); rschmidt1@unl.edu (R.J.S.)

[2] Department of Health, Exercise Science, and Recreation Management, University of Mississippi, Oxford, MS 38677, USA; bucknersamuel@gmail.com

[3] Department of Kinesiology and Health Promotion, University of Kentucky, Lexington, KY 40506-0219, USA; hbergstrom@uky.edu

* Correspondence: Nathaniel.jenkins@unl.edu (N.D.M.J.); jcramer@unl.edu (J.T.C.); Tel.: +1-402-472-7533 (J.T.C.)

Academic Editor: Lee E. Brown

Received: 18 August 2015; Accepted: 22 September 2015; Published: 25 September 2015

Abstract: This study compared electromyographic (EMG) amplitude, the number of repetitions completed, and exercise volume during three sets to failure of high- (80% 1RM) *versus* low-load (30% 1RM) forearm flexion resistance exercise on a subject-by-subject basis. Fifteen men were familiarized, completed forearm flexion 1RM testing. Forty-eight to 72 h later, the subjects completed three sets to failure of dumbbell forearm flexion resistance exercise with 80% ($n = 8$) or 30% ($n = 7$) 1RM. EMG amplitude was calculated for every repetition, and the number of repetitions performed and exercise volume were recorded. During sets 1, 2, and 3, one of eight subjects in the 80% 1RM group demonstrated a significant linear relationship for EMG amplitude *versus* repetition. For the 30% 1RM group, seven, five, and four of seven subjects demonstrated significant linear relationships during sets 1, 2, and 3, respectively. The mean EMG amplitude responses show that the fatigue-induced increases in EMG amplitude for the 30% 1RM group and no change in EMG amplitude for the 80% 1RM group resulted in similar levels of muscle activation in both groups. The numbers of repetitions completed were comparatively greater, while exercise volumes were similar in the 30% *versus* 80% 1RM group. Our results, in conjunction with those of previous studies in the leg extensors, suggest that there may be muscle specific differences in the responses to high- *versus* low-load exercise.

Keywords: electromyography; skeletal muscle; muscle fatigue; resistance training intensity; biceps brachii

1. Introduction

The current American College of Sports Medicine [1] and National Strength and Conditioning Association [2] guidelines recommend the utilization of resistance exercise loads corresponding to 60%–80% and 67%–85% of one repetition maximum (1RM), respectively, to maximize muscle hypertrophy. However, recent studies have challenged these recommendations [3–5]. For example, Burd *et al.* [3] demonstrated that acute resistance exercise performed to failure at 30% 1RM resulted in similar magnitudes of muscle protein synthesis and anabolic signaling as resistance exercise at 90% 1RM. In a follow-up study, Mitchell *et al.* [4] demonstrated that 10 weeks of leg extension resistance training to failure at 80% 1RM *versus* 30% 1RM resulted in comparable muscle hypertrophy. Similarly, Ogasawara *et al.* [5] showed that six weeks of bench press resistance training at 80% 1RM caused muscle hypertrophy equivalent to that observed after training at 30% 1RM. Therefore, the disparity between current resistance training recommendations and recent experimental results [3–5] has sparked a debate [6,7] regarding the most effective loads to prescribe to enhance muscle size with resistance training.

It has been suggested [8] that the recommendation of high-load resistance training (*i.e.*, ≥60% 1RM) to maximize muscle strength and hypertrophy is based on Henneman's size principle [9], which states that the recruitment of high-threshold motor units is dependent on the intensity of the stimulus [9]. Theoretically, therefore, motor unit recruitment is greater during resistance exercise at 80% 1RM than at 30% 1RM. While this may hold true for a single repetition in unfatigued muscle, the performance of submaximal contractions to volitional exhaustion may evoke the recruitment of additional motor units [10]. Accordingly, Burd *et al.* hypothesized that the similar acute increases in muscle protein synthesis and similar chronic muscle hypertrophy following low-load resistance training may be due to achieving "a similar degree of muscle fiber activation to that of high-intensity resistance exercise regimes." [11] (pp. 552–553). Burd *et al.* also suggested that the volume of exercise is "related to the degree of (muscle) fiber activation." [3] (pp. 7–8). However, while studies have examined muscle activation [12–15] and exercise volume [12] during high- *versus* low-load leg extension resistance exercise, we are unaware of previous studies that have compared muscle activation or exercise volume during high- *versus* low-load forearm flexion (*i.e.*, biceps curl) resistance exercise. Therefore, the purpose of this study was to compare electromyographic (EMG) amplitude, the number of repetitions completed, and exercise volume during three sets to failure of high- (80% 1RM) *versus* low-load (30% 1RM) forearm flexion resistance exercise on a subject-by-subject basis.

2. Materials and Methods

2.1. Subjects

Fifteen men (mean ± SD; age = 21.7 ± 2.4 years; height = 181.6 ± 7.5 cm; weight = 84.7 ± 23.5 kg) completed this study. Prior to any data collection, all subjects signed an informed consent form and completed a health history questionnaire. To be eligible, each participant must have been between the ages of 19 and 29, free from any current or ongoing musculoskeletal injuries or neuromuscular disorders involving the shoulders, elbows, or wrists, and could not have completed any regular or formal resistance training for at least six months prior to the start of the study. This study was approved by the university's Institutional Review Board for the protection of human subjects (IRB Approval #: 20140314046FB).

2.2. Experimental Design

A between-subjects design was utilized for this study, which consisted of three visits to the laboratory. During visits 1 and 2, subjects were familiarized with the exercises and procedures and forearm flexion (*i.e.*, biceps curl) 1RM was determined. The subjects were then randomized to either a high-load (80% 1RM; *n* = 8) or a low-load (30% 1RM; *n* = 7) resistance exercise group before returning to the laboratory 48 to 72 h later. During visit 3, subjects completed three sets to failure of bilateral dumbbell forearm flexion (e.g., biceps curl) resistance exercise with their assigned load. Each laboratory visit occurred at the same time of day (±2 h).

2.3. One Repetition Maximum

1RM testing was carried out according to the guidelines established by the National Strength and Conditioning Association [2]. Specifically, the subjects performed a light warm-up set with 5–10 repetitions at 50% of estimated 1RM, followed by 2–3 heavier warm-up sets of 2–5 repetitions with loads increasing by 10%–20% at each set. Subjects then began completing trials of 1 repetition with increasing loads (10%–20%) until they were no longer able to complete a single repetition. The highest load (kg) successfully lifted through the entire range of motion with the right arm with proper technique was denoted as the 1RM, which was determined in ≤4 trials for all subjects. Two to four min of rest were allowed between successive warm-up sets and 1RM trials. EMG and electrogoniometer signals were recorded from the right arm during the 1RM attempts.

2.4. Resistance Exercise

Subjects completed 3 sets of dumbbell forearm flexion resistance exercise to failure with loads corresponding (to the nearest 1.1 kg) to either 80% or 30% of 1RM. The subjects stood with their backs against a wall and their elbows supported by a brace (Bicep Bomber, Body Solid, Inc., Forest Park, IL, USA) to eliminate swinging of the torso or arms. Subjects were instructed to perform all repetitions through a complete range of motion. A metronome (Pro Metronome, EUMLab, Berlin, Germany) was set to 1 Hz, and participants were instructed to perform the concentric and eccentric phases corresponding with each tick of the metronome so that the concentric and eccentric phases were approximately 1 s. Verbal instruction and encouragement were provided during each set. Failure was defined as the inability to complete another concentric muscle action through the full range of motion. Two minutes of rest was provided between all sets for both groups. EMG and electrogoniometer signals were recorded from the right arm during all sets. In addition, the number of repetitions completed during each set was recorded and exercise volume was calculated as the product of the load (kg) and the number of repetitions completed during each set, summed across sets.

2.5. Electromyography

Pre-gelled bipolar surface electrodes (Ag/AgCl, AccuSensor, Lynn Medical, Wixom, MI, USA) were placed on the biceps brachii (BB) muscle of the right arm with an inter-electrode distance of 30 mm. The center of the bipolar electrode pair was placed at 33% of the distance between the fossa cubit and the medial acromion process [16]. A single pre-gelled surface electrode (Ag/AgCl, AccuSensor, Lynn Medical, Wixom, MI, USA) was placed on the lateral epicondyle of the humerus to serve as the reference electrode. To reduce inter-electrode impedance and increase the signal-to-noise ratio [17], local areas of the skin were shaved, abraded, and cleaned with isopropyl alcohol prior to the placement of the electrodes. Interelectrode impedance was kept below 2000 Ω [17].

2.6. Signal Processing

The EMG and goniometer signals were sampled at 2 kHz (MP150WSW, Biopac Systems, Inc., Santa Barbara, CA, USA), recorded on a personal computer, and processed off-line with custom software (Labview 12.0, National Instruments, Austin, TX, USA). The EMG signals were amplified (gain 1000) using a differential amplifier (EMG 100, Biopac Systems, Inc., Santa Barbara, CA, USA, bandwidth 1–5000 Hz) with a common mode rejection ratio of 110 dB min and an impedance of 2M Ω, digitally filtered (zero-phase shift 4th-order Butterworth filter) with a band-pass of 10–499 Hz, and rectified. The electrogoniometer signals were low-pass filtered (zero-phase shift 4th-order Butterworth filter) with a 15 Hz cutoff. The EMG amplitude was calculated as the time-averaged, integrated amplitude value ($\mu V \cdot s^{-1}$). EMG amplitude was quantified during the same 70° concentric portion of each repetition during each set, and then normalized to 1RM (expressed % 1RM). In addition, we compared EMG amplitude during the final common repetitions of sets 1, 2, and 3 for the 80% and 30% 1RM groups. The number of repetitions analyzed at the end of each set was established by the minimum number of repetitions achieved by any one subject within each group during sets 1, 2, and 3 (Table 1).

2.7. Statistics

Simple linear regression analyses were used to determine whether the slope coefficients for the individual EMG amplitude *versus* repetition relationships during sets 1, 2, and 3 were significantly different from zero. A type-I error rate of 5% was considered statistically significant for the linear regression analyses. Where applicable, 95% confidence intervals were calculated using the studentized t-distribution.

Table 1. The number of repetitions completed during sets 1, 2, and 3 and the volume (reps × load) completed across all sets, for each subject, as well as the mean (±95% confidence interval) volume completed for each group.

Group	Subject	Repetitions Completed			Individual Volume	Mean Volume
		Set 1	Set 2	Set 3	All sets	
80% 1RM	1	11	9	6	339.7	
	5	12	8	6	294.8	
	6	7	7	6	344.7	
	9	10	7	4	190.5	350.8 ± 72.8
	10	10	6	2	367.4	
	13	12	11	8	492.2	
	14	15	10	8	411.6	
	18	12	8	3	365.1	
30% 1RM	2	58	24	26	269.4	
	3	37	24	14	323.2	
	4	39	20	20	308.2	
	7	47	16	15	398.0	382.8 ± 101.4
	11	54	14	14	390.5	
	12	37	20	20	384.2	
	15	51	28	20	606.2	

3. Results

Table 1 displays the number of repetitions completed for each subject during each set, the total volume completed by each subject, and the mean (±95% confidence interval) volume completed by the 80% and 30% 1RM groups. The individual EMG amplitude *versus* repetition relationships for each subject during sets 1, 2, and 3 are depicted in Figure 1.

The results from the individual simple linear regression analyses for the EMG amplitude *versus* repetition relationships during sets 1, 2, 3 are depicted in Table 2. During sets 1, 2, and 3, one of eight subjects in the 80% 1RM group demonstrated a significant linear relationship. However, for the 30% 1RM group, seven of seven, five of seven, and four of seven subjects demonstrated significant linear relationships.

Figure 2 displays the EMG amplitude during the final common repetitions of sets 1, 2, and 3 for the 80% and 30% 1RM groups.

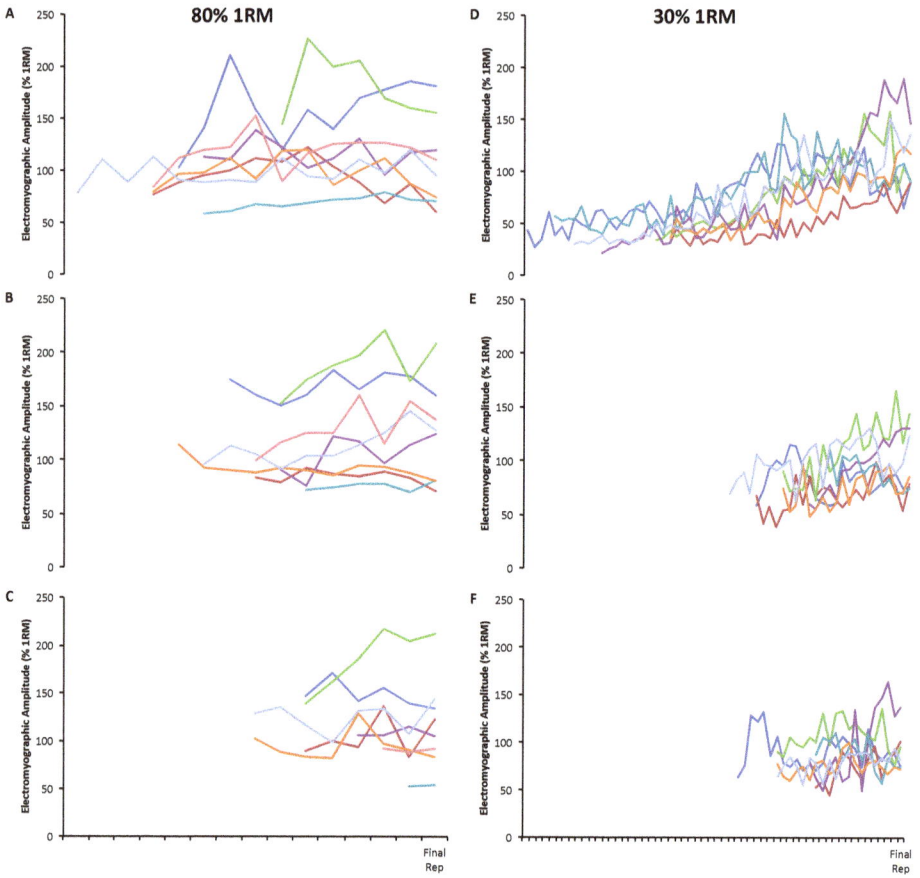

Figure 1. Individual electromyographic amplitude responses to resistance exercise at 80% one repetition maximum (1RM) during (**A**) set 1; (**B**) set 2; and (**C**) set 3 and at 30% 1RM during (**D**) set 1; (**E**) set 2; and (**F**) set 3.

Table 2. The individual simple linear regression analyses for the electromyographic (EMG) amplitude *versus* repetition relationships during sets 1, 2, and 3.

Group	Subject	Set 1				Set 2				Set 3			
		r	r^2	SEE	p-value	r	r^2	SEE	p-value	r	r^2	SEE	p-value
80% 1RM	1	0.50	0.25	28.36	0.11	0.24	0.06	12.11	0.54	0.58	0.34	12.13	0.23
	5	0.31	0.10	18.10	0.32	0.34	0.12	6.60	0.41	0.41	0.17	21.36	0.42
	6	0.32	0.10	31.90	0.48	0.66	0.44	19.08	0.11	0.90	0.82	14.95	0.01 *
	9	0.10	0.01	13.04	0.79	0.66	0.43	15.29	0.11	0.16	0.03	5.31	0.84
	10	0.84	0.71	3.56	<0.01 *	0.40	0.16	4.58	0.44	1.00	-	-	-
	13	0.08	0.01	15.80	0.80	0.59	0.35	6.95	0.05	0.07	<0.01	16.81	0.88
	14	0.33	0.11	11.80	0.23	0.77	0.59	11.09	<0.01 *	0.11	0.01	16.86	0.79
	18	0.28	0.08	17.90	0.37	0.66	0.43	16.71	0.08	0.06	<0.01	3.18	0.96
30% 1RM	2	0.76	0.58	16.70	<0.01 *	0.18	0.03	16.18	0.39	0.13	0.02	18.76	0.52
	3	0.85	0.73	9.12	<0.01 *	0.52	0.27	12.89	<0.01 *	0.66	0.44	13.35	0.01 *
	4	0.88	0.77	16.84	<0.01 *	0.80	0.64	16.91	<0.01 *	0.12	0.02	17.09	0.60
	7	0.90	0.80	21.50	<0.01 *	0.98	0.95	5.85	<0.01 *	0.77	0.59	26.43	<0.01 *
	11	0.76	0.58	19.26	<0.01 *	0.53	0.28	12.49	0.05	0.61	0.37	13.42	0.02 *
	12	0.92	0.84	10.26	<0.01 *	0.48	0.23	14.22	0.03 *	0.22	0.05	9.90	0.35
	15	0.93	0.86	12.91	<0.01 *	0.51	0.26	16.01	<0.01 *	0.50	0.25	9.72	0.03 *

r = correlation coefficient; r^2 = coefficient of determination; SEE = standard error of the estimate; * Indicates a significant relationship.

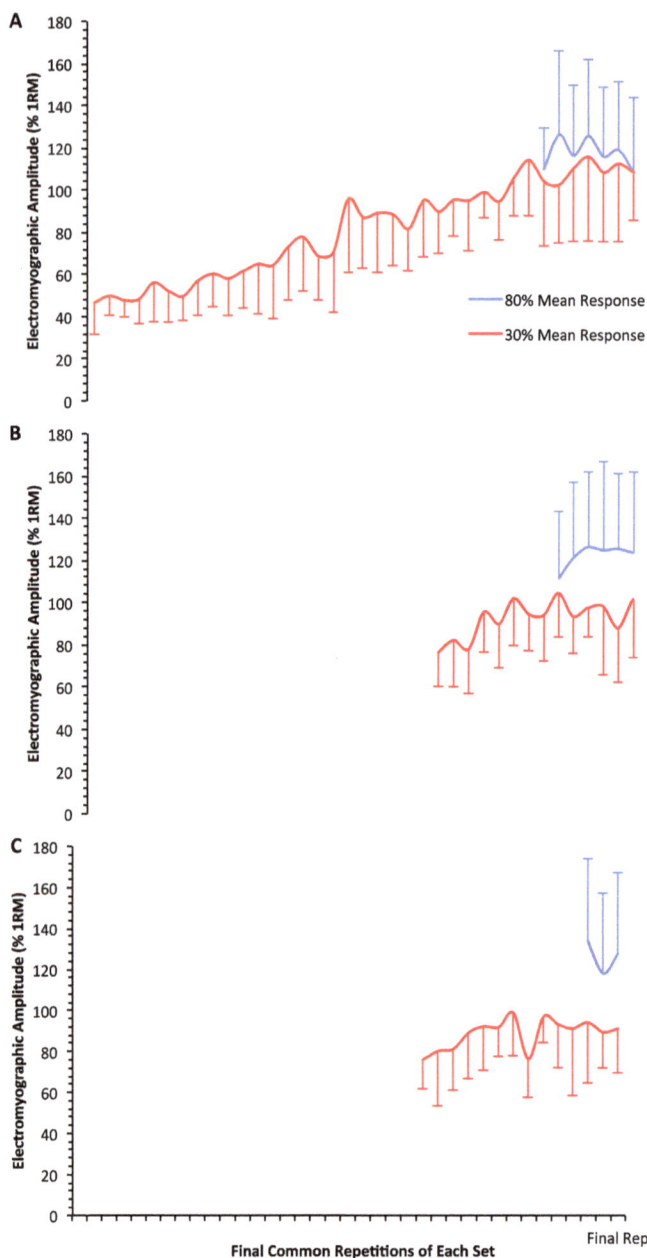

Figure 2. A comparison of the mean (±95% confidence interval) electromyographic amplitude responses during the final common repetitions for the 80% *versus* 30% 1RM groups during (**A**) set 1; (**B**) set 2; and (**C**) set 3. The number of repetitions analyzed for each set was based on the minimum number of repetitions achieved by any one subject in each group during sets 1, 2, and 3. For set 3, subject 10 was not included because he only completed two repetitions (see Table 1 for the repetitions completed by each subject during sets 1, 2, and 3).

4. Discussion

Mitchell *et al.* hypothesized that, "as lighter loads are repeated, the point of failure/fatigue ultimately necessitates near maximal motor unit recruitment to sustain muscle tension. Thus, relatively lighter loads lifted to the point of failure would result in a similar amount of muscle fiber activation compared with heavier loads lifted to failure" [4] (p. 75). Interestingly, our results supported this hypothesis [4]. The individual EMG amplitude *versus* repetition responses in our study indicated that muscle activation increased linearly for all subjects in the 30% 1RM group during set 1. Subsequently, however, EMG amplitude increased for five of seven and four of seven subjects during sets 2 and 3, respectively. In contrast, only one of eight subjects demonstrated an increase in EMG amplitude during the 80% 1RM group during sets 1, 2, and 3, which suggested that muscle activation started and remained at or near the same level across all repetitions and sets at 80% 1RM. Furthermore, the mean EMG amplitude responses (Figure 2) show that the fatigue-induced increases in EMG amplitude for the 30% 1RM group and no change in EMG amplitude for the 80% 1RM group resulted in similar levels of muscle activation in both groups. These results are in contrast to our recent study [12] and others [13,15,18] showing that muscle activation was higher during high- *versus* low-load leg extension resistance exercise to failure. The primary difference between the present study and those previous studies [12,13,15,18] is the muscle group studied. Factors such as location (*i.e.*, upper- *versus* lower-body), blood flow [19], architecture (*i.e.*, pennate *versus* fusiform), or fiber type composition [20,21] of the muscle may influence the activation responses to high- *versus* low-load resistance exercise. Therefore, the muscle activation achieved during high- compared to low-load resistance exercise to failure may be muscle specific.

The information provided by the amplitude of the surface EMG signal is considered a global measure of muscle activation [22]. Because traditional surface EMG is unable to isolate individual motor units, EMG amplitude is related to net motor unit activity, which is a function of both motor unit recruitment and motor unit firing rate [17,22]. Furthermore, EMG amplitude is influenced by peripheral (*i.e.*, fiber membranes properties, action potential shapes, *etc.*) factors [17,22]. Therefore, it is not possible to distinguish between alterations in motor unit recruitment and firing rate in the present study with EMG amplitude alone. However, the amplitude and frequency content of the surface mechanomyogram (MMG) are thought to reflect motor unit recruitment and global motor unit firing rate, respectively [23,24]. Therefore, future studies should examine the surface MMG signal in conjunction with surface EMG during high- *versus* low-load resistance exercise to failure to provide more specific information regarding changes in motor unit recruitment *versus* motor unit firing rate.

In the present study, the numbers of repetitions completed by the subjects in the 30% 1RM group were comparatively greater than the numbers completed by those in the 80% 1RM group (Table 1). This supports data presented by Jenkins *et al.* [12] who reported that the mean ± standard deviation for the numbers of repetitions completed during leg extension resistance training at 80% and 30% 1RM during sets 1, 2, and 3 were 8.9 ± 2.7 and 45.6 ± 14.3, 6.7 ± 1.9 and 26.8 ± 8.3, and 6.2 ± 1.7 and 22.2 ± 8.6 repetitions, respectively. Unexpectedly, however, the exercise volumes for the 80% and 30% 1RM groups were similar in the present study (Table 1). Previously, Jenkins *et al.* [12] showed that exercise volume during three sets of 30% 1RM leg extension resistance exercise was 58% greater than during three sets at 80% 1RM. Therefore, the volume of exercise performed during high- *versus* low-load training may be also be dependent on the muscle group studied, such that the exercise volume may be similar for high- and low-load exercise for the forearm flexors, but greater during low-load exercise for the leg extensors.

5. Conclusions

Overall, the results of the present study indicated that forearm flexion resistance exercise to failure at 30% 1RM caused fatigue-induced increases in EMG amplitude, whereas during 80% 1RM, EMG amplitude remained relatively constant (Figure 1). This load-dependent interaction for EMG amplitude led to similar levels of muscle activation during the final common repetitions at 80% and 30% 1RM

Sports **2015**, *3*, 269–280

(Figure 2). In addition, the numbers of repetitions achieved were comparatively greater for the 30% 1RM than the 80% 1RM group during sets 1, 2, and 3, while total exercise volume was similar between groups (Table 1). Thus, our results conflict with several previous studies [12,13,15,18] showing that muscle activation is greater, but exercise volume is lower [12], during 80% *versus* 30% 1RM resistance exercise in the leg-extensors. Future studies are needed with simultaneous examinations of EMG and MMG amplitude to better understand the interactions between motor unit recruitment and motor unit firing rate during these loading schemes. Based on the results of the present study, in conjunction with those of previous studies [12,13,15,18], the muscle activation responses and exercise volume completed during low-load training may be dependent on the location, blood flow, architecture, or fiber type composition of the muscle group studied.

Acknowledgments: The authors would like to thank Noelle M. Yeo and Jessie M. Miller for their help with data collection. This study was supported in part by the University of Nebraska Agricultural Research Division with funds provided through the Hatch Act (Agency: United States Department of Agriculture, National Institute of Food and Agriculture; Accession No: 1000080; Project No: NEB-36-078).

Author Contributions: Nathaniel D. M. Jenkins was the primary manuscript writer, and carried out data acquisition, data analysis, and data interpretation. Samuel L. Buckner, Haley C. Bergstrom, Kristen C. Cochrane, Cory M. Smith and Ethan C. Hill were significant contributors to data acquisition, read and approved the final manuscript, and were manuscript reviewers/revisers. Terry J. Housh and Richard J. Schmidt were significant manuscript reviewers/revisers. Joel T. Cramer was the primary manuscript reviewer/reviser, a substantial contributor to concept and design, and contributed to data analysis and interpretation.

Conflicts of Interest: The authors declare no conflict of interest.

References

1. Garber, C.E.; Blissmer, B.; Deschenes, M.R.; Franklin, B.A.; Lamonte, M.J.; Lee, I.M.; Nieman, D.C.; Swain, D.P. American college of sports medicine position stand. Quantity and quality of exercise for developing and maintaining cardiorespiratory, musculoskeletal, and neuromotor fitness in apparently healthy adults: Guidance for prescribing exercise. *Med. Sci. Sports Exerc.* **2011**, *43*, 1334–1359. [CrossRef] [PubMed]
2. National Strength and Conditioning Association. *Essentials of Strength Training and Conditioning*, 3rd ed.; Human Kinetics: Champaign, IL, USA, 2008.
3. Burd, N.A.; West, D.W.; Staples, A.W.; Atherton, P.J.; Baker, J.M.; Moore, D.R.; Holwerda, A.M.; Parise, G.; Rennie, M.J.; Baker, S.K.; *et al.* Low-load high volume resistance exercise stimulates muscle protein synthesis more than high-load low volume resistance exercise in young men. *PLoS ONE* **2010**, *5*. [CrossRef] [PubMed]
4. Mitchell, C.J.; Churchward-Venne, T.A.; West, D.W.; Burd, N.A.; Breen, L.; Baker, S.K.; Phillips, S.M. Resistance exercise load does not determine training-mediated hypertrophic gains in young men. *J. Appl. Physiol.* **2012**, *113*, 71–77. [CrossRef] [PubMed]
5. Ogasawara, R.; Loenneke, J.P.; Thiebaud, R.S.; Abe, T. Low-load bench press training to fatigue results in muscle hypertrophy similar to high-load bench press training. *Int. J. Clin. Med.* **2013**, *4*, 114–121. [CrossRef]
6. Burd, N.A.; Moore, D.R.; Mitchell, C.J.; Phillips, S.M. Big claims for big weights but with little evidence. *Eur. J. Appl. Physiol.* **2013**, *113*, 267–268. [CrossRef] [PubMed]
7. Schuenke, M.D.; Herman, J.; Staron, R.S. Preponderance of evidence proves "big" weights optimize hypertrophic and strength adaptations. *Eur. J. Appl. Physiol.* **2013**, *113*, 269–271. [CrossRef] [PubMed]
8. Carpinelli, R.N. The size principle and a critical analysis of the unsubstantiated heavier-is-better recommendation for resistance training. *J. Exerc. Sci. Fit.* **2008**, *6*, 67–86.
9. Henneman, E.; Somjen, G.; Carpenter, D.O. Functional significance of cell size in spinal motoneurons. *J. Neurophysiol.* **1965**, *28*, 560–580. [PubMed]
10. Conwit, R.A.; Stashuk, D.; Suzuki, H.; Lynch, N.; Schrager, M.; Metter, E.J. Fatigue effects on motor unit activity during submaximal contractions. *Arch. Phys. Med. Rehabil.* **2000**, *81*, 1211–1216. [CrossRef] [PubMed]
11. Burd, N.A.; Mitchell, C.J.; Churchward-Venne, T.A.; Phillips, S.M. Bigger weights may not beget bigger muscles: Evidence from acute muscle protein synthetic responses after resistance exercise. *Appl. Physiol. Nutr. Metab.* **2012**, *37*, 551–554. [CrossRef] [PubMed]

12. Jenkins, N.D.; Housh, T.J.; Bergstrom, H.C.; Cochrane, K.C.; Hill, E.C.; Smith, C.M.; Johnson, G.O.; Schmidt, R.J.; Cramer, J.T. Muscle activation during three sets to failure at 80% *vs.* 30% 1rm resistance exercise. *Eur. J. Appl. Physiol.* **2015**, in press. [CrossRef] [PubMed]

13. Akima, H.; Saito, A. Activation of quadriceps femoris including vastus intermedius during fatiguing dynamic knee extensions. *Eur. J. Appl. Physiol.* **2013**, *113*, 2829–2840. [CrossRef] [PubMed]

14. Schoenfeld, B.J. Potential mechanisms for a role of metabolic stress in hypertrophic adaptations to resistance training. *Sports Med.* **2013**, *43*, 179–194. [CrossRef] [PubMed]

15. Cook, S.B.; Murphy, B.G.; Labarbera, K.E. Neuromuscular function after a bout of low-load blood flow-restricted exercise. *Med. Sci. Sports Exerc.* **2013**, *45*, 67–74. [CrossRef] [PubMed]

16. Hermens, H.J.; Freriks, B.; Merletti, R.; Stegeman, D.; Blok, J.; Rau, G.; Disselhorst-Klug, C.; Hagg, G. *Seniam 8: European Recommendations for Surface Electromyography*; Roessngh Research and Development: Enschede, The Netherlands, 1999.

17. Beck, T.W.; Housh, T.J. Use of electromyography in studying human movement. In *Routledge Handbook of Biomechanics and Human Movement*; Hong, Y., Bartlett, R., Eds.; Routledge: New York, NY, USA, 2008; pp. 214–230.

18. Schoenfeld, B.J.; Contreras, B.; Willardson, J.M.; Fontana, F.; Tiryaki-Sonmez, G. Muscle activation during low- *versus* high-load resistance training in well-trained men. *Eur. J. Appl. Physiol.* **2014**, *114*, 2491–2497. [CrossRef] [PubMed]

19. Samanek, M.; Goetzova, J.; Fiserova, J.; Skovranek, J. Differences in muscle blood flow in upper and lower extremities of patients after correction of coarctation of the aorta. *Circulation* **1976**, *54*, 377–381. [CrossRef] [PubMed]

20. Ali, A.; Sundaraj, K.; Badlishah Ahmad, R.; Ahamed, N.U.; Islam, A.; Sundaraj, S. Muscle fatigue in the three heads of the triceps brachii during a controlled forceful hand grip task with full elbow extension using surface electromyography. *J. Hum. Kinet.* **2015**, *46*, 69–76. [CrossRef] [PubMed]

21. Harwood, B.; Dalton, B.H.; Power, G.A.; Rice, C.L. Motor unit properties from three synergistic muscles during ramp isometric elbow extensions. *Exp. Brain Res.* **2013**, *231*, 501–510. [CrossRef] [PubMed]

22. Farina, D.; Merletti, R.; Enoka, R.M. The extraction of neural strategies from the surface emg. *J. Appl. Physiol.* **2004**, *96*, 1486–1495. [CrossRef] [PubMed]

23. Beck, T.W.; Housh, T.J.; Cramer, J.T.; Weir, J.P.; Johnson, G.O.; Coburn, J.W.; Malek, M.H.; Mielke, M. Mechanomyographic amplitude and frequency responses during dynamic muscle actions: A comprehensive review. *Biomed. Eng. Online* **2005**, *4*. [CrossRef] [PubMed]

24. Gordon, G.; Holbourn, A.H. The sounds from single motor units in a contracting muscle. *J. Physiol.* **1948**, *107*, 456–464. [CrossRef] [PubMed]

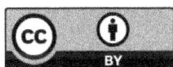

sports

MDPI

Article

Effectiveness of Different Rest Intervals Following Whole-Body Vibration on Vertical Jump Performance between College Athletes and Recreationally Trained Females

Nicole C. Dabbs [1,*], Jon A. Lundahl [2,†] and John C. Garner [2,†]

[1] Biomechanics and Sport Performance Laboratory, Department of Kinesiology, California State University, San Bernardino, 5500 University Parkway, San Bernardino, CA 92407, USA
[2] Applied Biomechanics Laboratory, Health, Exercise Science, and Recreation Management Department; The University of Mississippi, P.O. Box 1848, Oxford, MS 38677, USA; jonludndahl@gmail.com (J.A.L.); jcgarner@olemiss.edu (J.C.G.)
* Correspondence: ndabbs@csusb.edu; Tel.: +1-909-537-7565; Fax: +1-909-537-7085
† These authors contributed equally to this work.

Academic Editor: Lee E. Brown
Received: 4 August 2015; Accepted: 15 September 2015; Published: 18 September 2015

Abstract: The purpose of this study was to evaluate the effect of different rest intervals following whole-body vibration on counter-movement vertical jump performance. Sixteen females, eight recreationally trained and eight varsity athletes volunteered to participate in four testing visits separated by 24 h. Visit one acted as a familiarization visit where subjects were introduced to the counter-movement vertical jump and whole-body vibration protocols. Visits 2–4 contained 2 randomized conditions. Whole-body vibration was administered in four bouts of 30 s with 30 s rest between bouts. During whole-body vibration subjects performed a quarter squat every 5 s, simulating a counter-movement vertical jump. Whole-body vibration was followed by three counter-movement vertical jumps with five different rest intervals between the vibration exposure and jumping. For a control condition, subjects performed squats with no whole-body vibration. There was a significant ($p < 0.05$) main effect for time for vertical jump height, peak power output, and relative ground reaction forces, where a majority of individuals max jump from all whole-body vibration conditions was greater than the control condition. There were significant ($p < 0.05$) group differences, showing that varsity athletes had a greater vertical jump height and peak power output compared to recreationally trained females. There were no significant ($p > 0.05$) group differences for relative ground reaction forces. Practitioners and/or strength and conditioning coaches may utilize whole-body vibration to enhance acute counter-movement vertical jump performance after identifying individuals optimal rest time in order to maximize the potentiating effects.

Keywords: rest time; counter-movement; warm-up; athletic women

1. Introduction

Identifying key variables in an athlete's performance is essential to improving athletic performance. It is common to use traditional training techniques, such as strength training, plyometrics, and weightlifting and it may be beneficial to incorporate non-traditional techniques to further enhance performance [1–3]. It has become increasingly popular to incorporate non-traditional training modalities such as, whole-body vibration (WBV) [4–8] to achieve performance enhancement.

Whole-body vibration uses a platform that oscillates, sending vibration to the whole body while standing on the platform. It has been shown to improve upper and lower body muscular activity in both trained and untrained individuals [7,9–16]. Previous research indicates WBV exposure at a moderate intensity is safe and effective in stimulating the neuromuscular system [4] and has been shown to induce non-voluntary muscle contractions [17]. Power output is a key variable for sports performance and previous research have shown an increase in power production by facilitation of an explosive strength effort [9,18,19] leading to augmentation of performance via muscular strength and motor function [20,21]. Bouts of WBV exposure have also been seen to improve sprinting and jumping performance [5,8,10,22,23], with little or no effort by the individuals [24]. Although many studies has shown positive effects, there are several studies have shown no performance enhancements following WBV [5,7,12,25–27], resulting in inconsistency in previous literature.

Warming up prior to any physical performance is highly recommended and a widely accepted and acknowledged practice. WBV is increasingly being utilized as a warm-up for its potentiating effects prior to performance [5,8,13,16,24,28,29], to prepare the body for active performance instead of traditional warm-up techniques [30–32]. Further, WBV has been used passively and/or combined with active movements due to its reported acute performance enhancing effects [5,8]. The acute lower body neuromuscular activation from WBV [22,33] may be beneficial in many power sports.

Numerous variables during WBV exposure can affect optimal performance outcomes such as frequency, amplitude, duration, rest intervals, platform type, and population tested [8,22,23,34]. Several combinations of these variables have been manipulated in previous research, attempting to identify optimal performance. Rest intervals, specifically, have been shown to effect performance outcomes, varying from too short of rest with possible over stimulation of the neuromuscular system or too long of rest with possible dissipating effects [8,22]. Therefore, to increase performance variables, optimal rest intervals are critical when utilizing whole-body vibration. Previous research have shown conflicting results using varying rest intervals following acute bouts of WBV, from immediately post to 10 min [5,8,10,12,22,23,35,36]. To our knowledge there is no current literature that has investigated this vibration protocol with these specific rest times comparing athletes *versus* non-athletes.

Therefore, the purpose of this study was to investigate the effect of different rest intervals following WBV on vertical jump (VJ) performance in female recreationally trained and varsity athletes. Identifying optimal rest intervals following WBV exposure is critical to maximize vertical jump performance in trained individuals. Additionally, identifying differences between female varsity athletes and recreationally trained females will allow conclusions to be made on the applications of WBV exposure to different trained populations.

2. Material and Methods

2.1. Subjects

Sixteen females, recreationally trained ($n = 8$, age: 22 ± 1 year, height: 162.87 ± 2.6 cm, body mass: 64.35 ± 4.64 kg) and varsity athletes ($n = 8$, age: 20 ± 1 year, height: 168.19 ± 7.73 cm, body mass: 61.35 ± 9.68 kg) volunteered to participate in four testing visits. The participants were selected randomly from responders to fliers distributed over the university campus, and by word-of mouth.

Participants who were recreationally trained were defined as individuals who within the last year participated in lower body strength and power activities about three times a week. Varsity athletes were defined as highly trained athletes currently on a Division I athletic team. Participants were asked to refrain from any physical activity 24 h prior to testing and were excluded if they reported any lower body orthopedic injury or musculoskeletal injury within the past year. Each visit was within plus or minus one hour from initial to all proceeding visits, separated by at least 24 h. Participants were asked to wear comfortable clothing and the same shoes for each visit. Diet and hydration were not recorded but participants were asked to keep fluid and food consistent throughout the duration of the study. Each subject read and signed a university Institutional Review Board approved informed consent form prior to participation.

2.2. Study Design

The purpose of the study was to investigate acute performance potentiation following WBV exposure as it might be used in a potentiation warm-up procedure. Therefore, this study used a mixed factor-repeated measures design by having subjects perform five different rest interval conditions and comparing VJ performance to a control condition without WBV in recreationally trained and varsity athletes. Rest intervals ranged from immediate post to four minutes post.

2.3. Procedures

Visit one served as a familiarization session, which included completing the informed consent, anthropometric measurements, familiarization with the countermovement vertical jump (CMVJ) and WBV protocol. During the familiarization session, each subject completed three CMVJ's to assess variability; if the three CMVJ's exceeded 5% difference in jump height, they were asked to return to the lab on a subsequent day to complete another three jumps until the criterion was met. Participants then performed six experimental conditions in three days with two conditions per day [23] separated by a 10 min rest period. This rest period was deemed sufficient since previous literature has shown that WBV is ineffective after 10 min of exposure [22]. The order in which the conditions were performed was randomized and days were separated by at least 24 h.

WBV was performed on an AIRadaptive (Power Plate, Inc.) vibration platform, which administered a tri-axial vibration frequency at 30 Hz [5,22] and an amplitude setting low (2–4 mm). WBV sessions entailed four bouts of 30 s [23] for a total of two minutes of vibration exposure with 30 s rest between bouts. During WBV, subjects performed quarter squats [23,37] every 5 s while also simulating the arm swing used in a CMJ's. Participants were instructed to step off the plate during the bouts of rest. Following WBV exposure subjects were instructed to walk quickly to the force plate (~ 15 feet) to complete their rest interval for that condition followed by the three CMVJ's.

One condition served as a control during which participants stood on the vibration platform with no vibration, completed the squatting protocol then immediately performed three CMVJ's. The other five conditions used rest intervals of either immediately post, 0.5 min, 1 min, 2 min, or 4 min followed by three CMVJ's [22]. In addition, each subjects max value during experimental conditions for each variable (vertical jump height, peak power output, relative ground reaction forces), regardless of rest interval, was analyzed as another condition, thereby making seven conditions overall.

During all conditions participants were instructed to begin with their arms at a 90-degree angle then perform a CMVJ to a self-selected depth with arm swing and jump as high and as explosively as possible. Fifteen seconds of rest separated each jump and all jumps were performed on an AMTI force plate (Advanced Mechanical Technology, Inc., Watertown, MA, USA). A Vertec® (Columbus, OH, USA) was used as a visual target and to measure jump height to the nearest half-inch and was positioned next to the force plate. Vertical jump height (VJH) was measured and peak power output (PPO) was calculated using the Sayers equation [38]. Peak relative ground reaction force (rGRF) was sampled at 1000 Hz and maximum values from the highest jump from each condition were used for analysis. After completing one condition subjects sat in a chair with no active movement for 10 min then completed the second condition for that visit.

2.4. Statistical Analyses

All statistical procedures were conducted using the Statistical Package for the Social Sciences (PASW 20.0 for Windows, SPSS, Inc., Chicago, IL, USA). An a-priori alpha was set at 0.05 to determine significance. Differences between groups for height, weight, and age were analyzed with a one-way ANOVA. Differences in VJH, Peak Power, and rGRF between conditions were analyzed with a 2×7 (training status by condition) mixed factor ANOVA.

3. Results

There were no significant differences between recreationally trained and athletes in height ($p = 0.08$), weight ($p = 0.44$), and age ($p = 0.07$). There was no significant interaction for training status and time for VJH ($p = 0.18$), PPO ($p = 0.18$), and rGRF ($p = 0.97$). There was a significant main effect for time for VJH ($p < 0.001$), PPO ($p < 0.001$), and rGRF ($p = 0.01$), where each individuals max jump from all WBV conditions was greater than the control condition (Figure 1), however no significant ($p > 0.05$) differences were found between all other conditions (Table 1). There was a significant group differences, showing that varsity athletes had a greater VJH ($p < 0.001$) and PPO ($p < 0.001$) compared to recreationally trained females. There were no significant ($p = 0.96$) group differences for rGRF (Figure 2). Additionally, where each participant reached their max jump during the experimental conditions is list here: IM = 4, 0.5 min = 2, 1 min = 3, 2 min = 6, and 4 min = 1.

Table 1. Vertical Jump Height (VJH), Peak Power Output (PPO), and relative ground reaction force (rGFR) maximum values and values for each condition (mean ± SD) for varsity athletes and recreationally trained.

Conditions	VJH (cm)		PPO (W)		rGRF (N)	
	Varsity	Rec	Varsity	Rec	Varsity	Rec
Control	50.48 ± 6.78	42.06 ± 5.74 *	4062.50 ± 411.54	3551.79 ± 348.27 *	1608.91 ± 510.74	1613.90 ± 356.66
0 min	50.95 ± 7.0	41.91 ± 4.55 *	4091.41 ± 425.11	3542.15 ± 276.42 *	1616.72 ± 502.40	1599.02 ± 363.28
5 min	51.91 ± 6.84	39.84 ± 5.72 *	4149.23 ± 415.01	3416.88 ± 347.05 *	1629.38 ± 561.86	1645.71 ± 327.41
1 min	48.89 ± 9.77	40.95 ± 6.29 *	3966.14 ± 592.85	3484.34 ± 381.57 *	1626.78 ± 468.27	1628.41 ± 289.14
2 min	50.16 ± 6.18	43.33 ± 2.29 *	4043.23 ± 375.40	3628.88 ± 145.32 *	1629.38 ± 525.42	1600.58 ± 384.68
4 min	50.80 ± 8.56	40.64 ± 6.40 *	4081.78 ± 519.59	3465.06 ± 388.73 *	1662.43 ± 634.03	1643.70 ± 387.99
Max	53.34 ± 7.25 #	44.45 ± 3.84 *#	4235.95 ± 439.96 #	3696.33 ± 233.10 *#	1727.36 ± 387.99 #	1692.04 ± 355.47 #

* indicates significant ($p < 0.05$) differences between varsity and recreational athletes; # indicates significant ($p < 0.05$) differences greater than control.

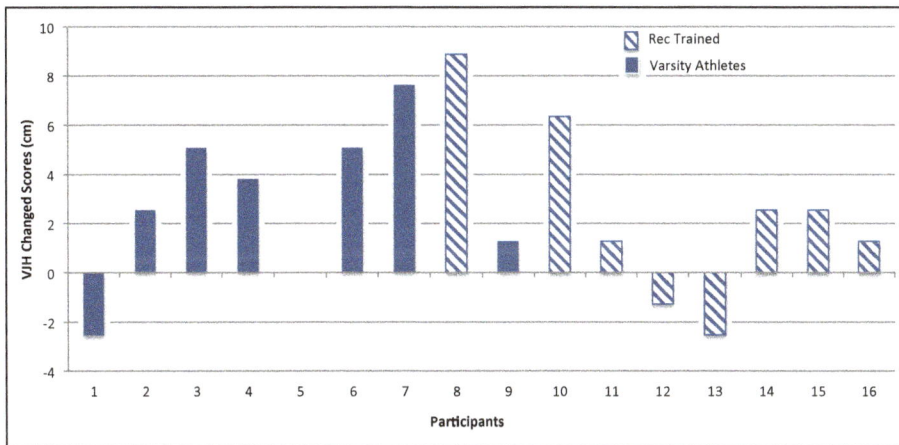

Figure 1. Individual differences between control and maximal VJ height (cm).

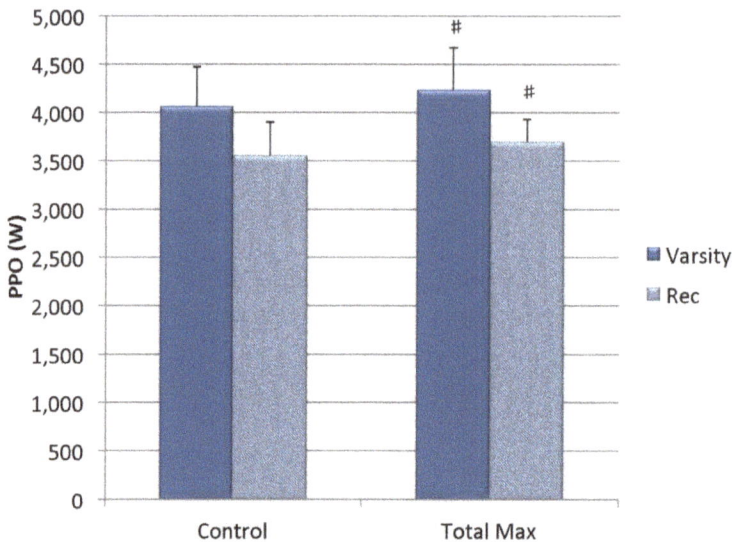

Figure 2. Differences between control condition and max condition for Peak Power Output (PPO) for varsity and recreationally trained females. # indicates significant ($p < 0.05$) differences between conditions; * indicates significant ($p < 0.05$) differences between groups.

4. Discussion

The aim of the current investigation was to determine the optimal rest interval following bouts of WBV on vertical jump performance variables. The main findings were that following WBV; VJH, PPO, and rGRF showed individual increases during one of the rest interval conditions with WBV exposure compared to the control condition (no WBV). Indicating that individuals respond differently to the WBV exposure, resulting in individual optimal rest times following WBV exposure. Another finding in this investigation was that for all conditions varsity female athletes had a greater VJH and PPO compared to the recreationally trained females.

In a previous study, the researchers found individual optimal rest intervals between WBV exposure and vertical jumping performance, similar to the current investigation using similar protocols but comparing recreationally trained males and females only [8] instead of an athletic population. These similarities indicate that regardless of training status or sex, a majority of individuals responded to the WBV exposure and had an increased vertical jump performance. The only other methodical difference from this particular previous research was that the current study used a tri-axial WBV platform, while the previous study used a pivotal vibration platform. Therefore, similar results in both studies indicate that the type of vibration platform exposure has similar benefits on vertical jump performance as well. This is a positive finding, since most research studies using WBV are done on a variety of platforms, it is often uncertain if researchers can make comparisons. Previous studies have examined the differences using different types of WBV platforms [34,39], since different platforms have different oscillatory motions. A recent study examined the differences in three platform types and found no differences on their acute vertical jump performance [34]. The researcher concluded that different devices could be used similarly for acute vertical jump performance bouts.

Other key variables are critical when using WBV for performance enhancement such as frequency, amplitude, rest times, and vibration exposure time. Frequency can easily be changed on most devices and can be described as the intensity of the vibration where amplitude can be described as the volume. Previous research has shown that 1 min rest post vibration exposure and a frequency of 30 Hz were optimal for vertical jump performance increases [22,23]. The frequency exposure was similar to the current study, however our study did differ in the time exposure of WBV. Bedient and Adams [22,23] exposed participants to one bout of 30 s of WBV and found an increase in CMVJ, resulting in a homogenous optimal rest interval of 1 min post when compared to immediate post, 5 min, or 10 min. In contrast, our study exposed subjects to four bouts of 30 s of vibration with a 1:1 rest ratio, and found individual optimal rest intervals for an increase in vertical jump performance. In contrast, another study examined varied frequencies and durations of vibration exposures and found no differences in vertical jump performance, indicating no conclusive frequency or vibration exposure time [34].

There are some research studies that conclude that using WBV prior to vertical jump performance induces a post-activation potentiation (PAP) response [5,35]. PAP has been shown to increase voluntary force development during muscle actions [40] but can induce fatigue if the intensity is too high or there is not sufficient rest periods before performance [41]. PAP has been shown to vary on an individual basis [42], some individuals have different optimal rest times and fatigue effects, which should be considered when inducing PAP [41]. Previous research that uses WBV for PAP to enhance vertical jump performance have seen positive effects at enhancing acute performance [5,8,35]. In the current investigation, no differences between rest intervals were found, however when taking individual max vertical jump values with WBV and comparing it to the control group, individuals showed an increase in vertical jump performance. Thus, the increases in vertical jump performance induced by WBV may have been sufficient enough to induce PAP but limited enough not to induce fatigue.

The current study compared female college athletes to recreationally trained females. As we expected, the college athletes performed at a higher level with greater vertical jump performance compared to the recreationally trained individuals. These results are most likely contributed to college athletes having a higher level of training, increasing their potential to develop a higher force generating capacity [42], resulting in a higher VJH. Additionally, the athletic population may have more experience with vertical jumping allowing them to have greater vertical jumping performance accompanied with a higher level of strength and conditioning periodized programs required by their college sport. However, there have been conflicting results in a variety of studies with athletic and recreationally trained individuals with WBV and jumping performance [7,8,43,44]. In the current study, there were no group differences in the rGRF but there was a difference for VJH and PPO. This may be due to the use of the Vertec® device to measure VJH instead of estimating flight time from the force plate. The use of the Vertec® doesn't account for changes in arm reach or trunk twist during the jumps, which may modify scores [45]. On the other hand, VJH estimation could be altered with landing mechanics when using the force plate [45].

Our study has a few potential limitations that may have influenced the results of our study. One may have been our testing protocol, there were two conditions performed in one testing day with a 10 min washout period between conditions. This was randomized to control for any learning effects however, it is possible that one condition influenced the other. Research suggests that after 10 min, WBV has no effect on vertical jump performance [22], therefore we do not suspect a learning effect occurred. Another limitation may have been that since our data reflects the maximum VJH for each condition, it is possible that it may have affected subsequent VJ performance. However, previous research shows that when analyzing kinetics during VJ performance there were no subsequent effects shown [46]. It is important to note that three of the participants actually perform better in the control condition compared to the experimental condition. This has been shown in other studies and has been suggested that there are responder and non-responders to WBV treatment [8]. Another important limitation to mention is the small power due to the sample size. A critical factor is the type of WBV platform utilized. The present study utilized a tri-axial platform where others [8,22,23,35] have utilized similar and other types (e.g., vertical, sliding horizontal, and pivotal), which may affect the outcome of the study.

Sports **2015**, *3*, 258–268

5. Conclusions

Post activation potentiation was induced using whole-body vibration exposure on vertical jump performance on eight female college athletes and eight recreationally trained females. Four sets of 30 s bouts of WBV prior to vertical jump performance showed statistically significant differences between individual maximum jumps at different rest times with WBV compared to the control (no WBV). Therefore, it is recommended that practitioners determine individual optimal rest times following WBV prior to high level performance to obtain greatest potentiating effects. Acquiring individual optimal rest times prior to performance would allow individuals to maximum their potentiating acute effects in a single explosive movement. Therefore, this study specifically applies to female athletes that perform single bouts of explosive movements such as, high jumpers and long jumpers. Once optimal rest time is determined, it will allow for optimal performance during competition. This investigation has shown these effects to be applied to female athletic and recreationally trained individuals.

Author Contributions: Nicole Dabbs, Jon Lundahl, and John Garner were involved in study design, data collection, data interpretation, and manuscript writing.

Conflicts of Interest: The authors declare no conflict of interest.

References

1. Kraemer, W.J.; Ratamess, N.A. Fundamentals of resistance training: Progression and exercise prescription. *Med. Sci. Sports Exerc.* **2004**, *36*, 674–688. [CrossRef] [PubMed]
2. Newton, R.U.; Gerber, A.; Nimphius, S.; Shim, J.K.; Doan, B.K.; Robertson, M.; Pearson, D.R.; Craig, B.W.; Häkkinen, K.; Kraemer, W.J. Determination of functional strength imbalance of the lower extremities. *J. Strength Cond. Res.* **2006**, *20*, 971–977. [PubMed]
3. Newton, R.U.; Kraemer, W.J.; Hakkinen, K. Effects of ballistic training on preseason preparation of elite volleyball players. *Med. Sci. Sports Exerc.* **1999**, *31*, 323–330. [CrossRef] [PubMed]
4. Cardinale, M.; Bosco, C. The use of vibration as an exercise intervention. *Exerc. Sport Sci. Rev.* **2003**, *31*, 3–7. [CrossRef] [PubMed]
5. Cormie, P.; Deane, R.S.; Triplett, N.T.; McBride, J.M. Acute effects of whole-body vibration on muscle activity, strength, and power. *J. Strength Cond. Res.* **2006**, *20*, 257–261. [PubMed]
6. Da Silva, M.E.; Fernandez, J.M.; Castillo, E.; Nuñez, V.M.; Vaamonde, D.M.; Poblador, M.S.; Lancho, J.L. Influence of vibration training on energy expenditure in active men. *J. Strength Cond. Res.* **2007**, *21*, 470–475. [PubMed]
7. Dabbs, N.C.; Brown, L.E.; Coburn, J.W.; Lynn, S.K.; Tran, T.T.; Biagini, M.S. Effect of Whole-body vibration warm-up on bat speed in women softball players. *J. Strength Cond. Res.* **2010**, *24*, 2296–2299. [CrossRef] [PubMed]
8. Dabbs, N.C.; Muñoz, C.X.; Tran, T.T.; Brown, L.E.; Bottaro, M. Effect of different rest intervals after whole-body vibration on vertical jump performance. *J. Strength Cond. Res.* **2011**, *25*, 662–667. [CrossRef] [PubMed]
9. Bosco, C.; Cardinale, M.; Tsarpela, O. Influence of vibration on mechanical power and electromyogram activity in human arm flexor muscles. *Eur. J. Appl. Physiol. Occup. Physiol.* **1999**, *79*, 306–311. [CrossRef] [PubMed]
10. Bullock, N.; Martin, D.T.; Ross, A.; Rosemond, C.D.; Jordan, M.J.; Marino, F.E. Acute effect of whole-body vibration on sprint and jumping performance in elite skeleton athletes. *J. Strength Cond. Res.* **2008**, *22*, 1371–1374. [CrossRef] [PubMed]
11. Cochrane, D.J.; Hawke, E.J. Effects of acute upper-body vibration on strength and power variables in climbers. *J. Strength Cond. Res.* **2007**, *21*, 527–531. [PubMed]
12. Cochrane, D.J.; Stannard, S.R. Acute whole body vibration training increases vertical jump and flexibility performance in elite female field hockey players. *Br. J. Sports Med.* **2005**, *39*, 860–865. [CrossRef] [PubMed]
13. Dallas, G.; Kirialanis, P.; Mellos, V. The acute effect of whole body vibration training on flexibility and explosive strength of young gymnasts. *Biol. Sport* **2014**, *31*, 233–237. [CrossRef] [PubMed]

14. Di Loreto, C.; Ranchelli, A.; Lucidi, P.; Murdolo, G.; Parlanti, N.; de Cicco, A.; Tsarpela, O.; Annino, G.; Bosco, C.; Santeusanio, F.; *et al.* Effects of whole-body vibration exercise on the endocrine system of healthy men. *J. Endocrinol. Investig.* **2004**, *27*, 323–327. [CrossRef] [PubMed]

15. Jacobs, P.L.; Burns, P. Acute enhancement of lower-extremity dynamic strength and flexibility with whole-body vibration. *J. Strength Cond. Res.* **2009**, *23*, 51–57. [CrossRef] [PubMed]

16. Despina, T.; George, D.; George, T.; Sotiris, P.; Alessandra, D.C.; George, K.; Maria, R.; Stavros, K. Short-term effects of whole-body vibration training on balance, flexibility and lower limb explosive strength in elite rhythmic gymnasts. *Hum. Mov. Sci.* **2014**, *33*, 149–158. [CrossRef] [PubMed]

17. Issurin, V.B. Vibrationss and their applications in sport: A review. *J. Sports Med. Phys. Fit.* **2005**, *45*, 424–436.

18. Issurin, V.B.; Tenenbaum, G. Acute and residual effects of vibratory stimulation on explosive strength in elite and amateur athletes. *J. Sports Sci.* **1999**, *17*, 177–182. [CrossRef] [PubMed]

19. Poston, B.; Holcomb, W.R.; Guadagnoli, M.A.; Linn, L.L. The acute effects of mechanical vibration on power output in the bench press. *J. Strength Cond. Res.* **2007**, *21*, 199–203. [CrossRef] [PubMed]

20. Bosco, C.; Cardinale, M.; Tsarpela, O.; Colli, R.; Tihanyi, J.; von Duvillard, S.P.; Viru, A. The influence of whole body vibration on jumping performance. *Biol. Sports.* **1998**, *15*, 157–614.

21. Bosco, C.; Colli, R.; Introini, E.; Cardinale, M.; Tsarpela, O.; Madella, A.; Tihanyi, J.; Viru, A. Adaptive responses of human skeletal muscle to vibration exposure. *Clin. Physiol.* **1999**, *19*, 183–187. [CrossRef] [PubMed]

22. Adams, J.B.; Edwards, D.; Serravite, D.H.; Bedient, A.M.; Huntsman, E.; Jacobs, K.A.; del Rossi, G.; Roos, B.A.; Signorile, J.F. Optimal frequency, displacement, duration, and recovery patterns to maximize power output following acute whole-body vibration. *J. Strength Cond. Res.* **2009**, *23*, 237–245. [CrossRef] [PubMed]

23. Bedient, A.M.; Adams, J.B.; Edwards, D.A.; Serravite, D.H.; Huntsman, E.; Mow, S.E.; Roos, B.A.; Signorile, J.F. Displacement and frequency for maximizing power output resulting from a bout of whole-body vibration. *J. Strength Cond. Res.* **2009**, *23*, 1683–1687. [CrossRef] [PubMed]

24. Rittweger, J.; Beller, G.; Felsenberg, D. Acute physiological effects of exhaustive whole-body vibration exercise in man. *Clin Physiol.* **2000**, *20*, 134–142. [CrossRef] [PubMed]

25. De Ruiter, C.J.; van der Linden, R.M.; van der Zijden, M.J.; Hollander, A.P.; de Haan, A. Short-term effects of whole-body vibration on maximal voluntary isometric knee extensor force and rate of force rise. *Eur. J. Appl. Physiol.* **2003**, *88*, 472–475. [CrossRef] [PubMed]

26. Kelly, S.B.; Alvar, B.A.; Black, L.E.; Dodd, D.J.; Carothers, K.F.; Brown, L.E. The effect of warm-up with whole-body vibration *vs.* cycle ergometry on isokinetic dynamometry. *J. Strength Cond. Res.* **2010**, *24*, 3140–3143. [CrossRef] [PubMed]

27. Menefee, K.; Switzler, C.; Podlog, L.; Hickes-Little, C. The acute effects of two different foot positions during whole body vibration on vertical jump performance in females. *J. Athl. Med.* **2014**, *2*, 66–74.

28. Cochrane, D.J.; Stannard, S.R.; Sargeant, A.J.; Rittweger, J. The rate of muscle temperature increase during acute whole-body vibration exercise. *Eur. J. Appl. Physiol.* **2008**, *103*, 441–448. [CrossRef] [PubMed]

29. Dallas, G.; Kirialanis, P. The effects of two different conditions of whole-body vibration on flexibility and jumping performance on artistic gymnasts. *Sci. Gymnast. J.* **2013**, *5*, 41–52.

30. Burkett, L.N.; Phillips, W.T.; Ziuraitis, J. The best warm-up for the vertical jump in college-age athletic men. *J. Strength Cond. Res.* **2005**, *19*, 673–676. [PubMed]

31. Chaouachi, A.; Castagna, C.; Chtara, M.; Brughelli, M.; Turki, O.; Galy, O.; Chamari, K.; Behm, D.G. Effect of warm-ups involving static or dynamic stretching on agility, sprinting, and jumping performance in trained individuals. *J. Strength Cond. Res.* **2010**, *24*, 2001–2011. [CrossRef] [PubMed]

32. Gourgoulis, V.; Aggeloussis, N.; Kasimatis, P.; Mavromatis, G.; Garas, A. Effect of a submaximal half-squats warm-up program on vertical jumping ability. *J. Strength Cond. Res.* **2003**, *17*, 342–344. [PubMed]

33. Abercromby, A.F.; Amonette, W.E.; Layne, C.S.; McFarlin, B.K.; Hinman, M.R.; Paloski, W.H. Variation in neuromuscular responses during acute whole-body vibration exercise. *Med. Sci. Sports Exerc.* **2007**, *39*, 1642–1650. [CrossRef] [PubMed]

34. Bagheri, J.; van den Berg-Emons, R.J.; Pel, J.J.; Horemans, H.L.; Stam, H.J. Acute effects of whole-body vibration on jump force and jump rate of force development: A comparative study of different devices. *J. Strength Cond. Res.* **2012**, *26*, 691–696. [CrossRef] [PubMed]

35. McBride, J.M.; Nuzzo, J.L.; Dayne, A.M.; Israetel, M.A.; Nieman, D.C.; Triplett, N.T. Effect of an acute bout of whole body vibration exercise on muscle force output and motor neuron excitability. *J. Strength Cond. Res.* **2010**, *24*, 184–189. [CrossRef] [PubMed]

36. Ronnestad, B.R. Acute effects of various whole-body vibration frequencies on lower-body power in trained and untrained subjects. *J. Strength Cond. Res.* **2009**, *23*, 1309–1315. [CrossRef] [PubMed]

37. Cochrane, D.J.; Legg, S.J.; Hooker, M.J. The short-term effects of whole-body vibration training on vertical jump, sprint, and agility performance. *J. Strength Cond. Res.* **2004**, *18*, 828–832. [PubMed]

38. Sayers, S.P.; Harackiewicz, D.V.; Harman, E.A.; Frykman, P.N.; Rosenstein, M.T. Cross-validation of three jump power equations. *Med. Sci. Sports Exerc.* **1999**, *31*, 572–577. [CrossRef] [PubMed]

39. Pel, J.J.; Bagheri, J.; van Dam, L.M.; van den Berg-Emons, H.J.; Horemans, H.L.; Stam, H.J.; van der Steen, J. Platform accelerations of three different whole-body vibration devices and the transmission of vertical vibrations to the lower limbs. *Med. Eng. Phys.* **2009**, *31*, 937–944. [CrossRef] [PubMed]

40. Tillin, N.; Bishop, D. Factors modulating post-activation potentiation and its effect on performance of subsequent explosive ativities. *Sports Med.* **2009**, *39*, 147–166. [CrossRef] [PubMed]

41. McCann, M.R.; Flanagan, S.P. The effects of exercise selection and rest interval on postactivation potentiation of vertical jump performance. *J. Strength Cond. Res.* **2010**, *24*, 1285–1291. [CrossRef] [PubMed]

42. Chiu, L.Z.; Fry, A.C.; Weiss, L.W.; Schilling, B.K.; Brown, L.E.; Smith, S.L. Postactivation potentiation response in athletic and recreationally trained individuals. *J. Strength Cond. Res.* **2003**, *17*, 671–677. [PubMed]

43. Burns, J.D.; Miller, P.C.; Hall, E.E. *Acute Effects of Whole Body Vibration on Functional Capabilities of Skeletal Muscle*; Federación Española de Asociaciones de Docentes de Educación Física: Elon, NC, USA, 2015; pp. 180–183.

44. Naclerio, F.; Faigenbaum, A.D.; Larumbe-Zabala, E.; Ratamess, N.A.; Kang, J.; Friedman, P.; Ross, R.E. Effectiveness of different postactivation potentiation protocols with and without whole body vibration on jumping performance in college athletes. *J. Strength Cond. Res.* **2014**, *28*, 232–239. [CrossRef] [PubMed]

45. Ferreira, L.C.; Schilling, B.K.; Weiss, L.W.; Fry, A.C.; Chiu, L.Z. Reach height and jump displacement: Implications for standardization of reach determination. *J. Strength Cond. Res.* **2010**, *24*, 1596–1601. [CrossRef] [PubMed]

46. Jensen, R.L.; Ebben, W.P. Kinetic analysis of complex training rest interval effect on vertical jump performance. *J. Strength Cond. Res.* **2003**, *17*, 345–349. [PubMed]

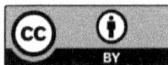

sports

MDPI

Communication

The Effect of Kettlebell Swing Load and Cadence on Physiological, Perceptual and Mechanical Variables

Michael J. Duncan *, Rosanna Gibbard, Leanne M. Raymond and Peter Mundy

Centre for Applied Biological and Exercise Sciences, Coventry University, Coventry CV11 5FB, UK;
gibbardr@uni.coventry.ac.uk (R.G.); raymondl@uni.coventry.ac.uk (L.M.R.); ab9674@coventry.ac.uk (P.M.)
* Correspondence: michael.duncan@coventry.ac.uk; Tel./Fax: 0044-247-688-613

Academic Editor: Lee E. Brown
Received: 16 July 2015; Accepted: 4 August 2015; Published: 7 August 2015

Abstract: This study compared the physiological, perceptual and mechanical responses to kettlebell swings at different loads and swing speeds. Following familiarization 16 strength trained participants (10 males, six females, mean age $\pm$ SD = 23 $\pm$ 2.9) performed four trials: 2 min kettlebell swings with an 8 kg kettlebell at a fast cadence; 2 min kettlebell swings with an 8 kg kettlebell at a slow cadence; 4 min kettlebell swings with a 4 kg kettlebell at a fast cadence; 4 min kettlebell swings with a 4 kg kettlebell at a slow cadence. Repeated measured analysis of variance indicated no significant differences in peak blood lactate or peak net vertical force across loads and cadences ($P > 0.05$). Significant main effect for time for heart rate indicated that heart rate was higher at the end of each bout than at mid-point ($P = 0.001$). A significant Load X cadence interaction for rating of perceived exertion (RPE) ($P = 0.030$) revealed that RPE values were significantly higher in the 8 kg slow cadence condition compared to the 4 kg slow ($P = 0.002$) and 4 kg fast ($P = 0.016$) conditions. In summary, this study indicates that the physiological and mechanical responses to kettlebell swings at 4 kg and 8 kg loads and at fast and slow cadence were similar, whereas the perceptual response is greater when swinging an 8 kg kettlebell at slow cadence.

Keywords: force; swing; nontraditional training; resistance exercise

---

1. Introduction

Kettlebells comprise a cast iron/steel weight, resembling a cannonball with a handle and are popular and widely used for resistance training. Their use has been advocated as a means to enhance muscular strength and endurance, and aerobic endurance whilst also reducing body fatness [1]. Unlike dumbbells, kettlebell training tends to comprise ballistic and swing movements where the centre of mass of the kettlebell is extended beyond the hand. Kettlebell training has also been recommended to condition occupation groups including the armed services [2] as well as being an efficacious rehabilitation tool [3,4]. While the use of the kettlebell dates back to circa 1700 s [1], scientific analysis of kettlebell training and individual movements with a kettlebell has only recently gathered momentum. Consequently, there are still significant gaps in the literature relating to the best use of kettlebells for strength and conditioning.

To date, studies examining kettlebell science have tended to focus on either physiological variables [5–7] or biomechanical variables [8,9]. A number of studies have also compared kettlebell exercise to treadmill running [7,10]. For example, Hulsey *et al.* [10] reported higher caloric expenditure, oxygen uptake (VO_2), metabolic equivalents and pulmonary ventilation during treadmill exercise, compared to 10 min kettlebell swinging. More recent work by Thomas *et al.* [7] compared a moderate-intensity kettlebell protocol with brisk walking performed on a treadmill. Ten novice participants performed a 30 min kettlebell protocol, comprising three continuous sets of 10 kettlebell swings followed by 10 sumo deadlifts (16 kg for males, 12 kg for females) with a 3 min rest between sets. This was compared to a 30 min treadmill walk (3,10 min bouts separated by 3 min rest) where VO_2 was matched from the kettlebell session. Their data indicated similar blood pressure, energy expenditure and respiratory exchange ratios between conditions but higher rating of perceived exertion (RPE) and heart rate during kettlebell exercise. Thomas *et al.* concluded that kettlebell training may therefore be used to enhance aerobic capacity to the same extent as brisk walking. Mechanically focused studies of kettlebell exercise have reported that kettlebell exercise results in a hip-hinge squat pattern, eliciting rapid muscle activation-relaxation cycles, opposite in polarity to that of traditional Olympic weightlifting techniques [9]. Other work [8] has reported on the mechanical demands of the kettlebell swing specifically. In their study, 16 males performed two sets of 10 kettlebell swings with 16, 24, and 32 kg kettlebells. Lake and Lauder [8] reported that swing mean and peak power was greater than power recorded during a back squat and comparable with power recorded from a jump squat.

A recent review of kettlebell research suggested a need to examine the effects of different kettlebell loads, as research has not fully examined responses across the range of kettlebell loads available [11]. Understanding the optimal loads for kettlebell training is an important consideration for coaches and athletes, yet without this initial comparison type research, this aspiration will not be elucidated. Moreover, in by far the majority of research using kettlebell training, participants have used different loads. For example, in Thomas *et al.* [7] kettlebell load differed between males and females, whereas in Lake and Lauder [8] participants performed two sets of 10 kettlebell swings across a standardised spectrum of kettlebell loads. As such, it is difficult to compare across kettlebell loads as the total volume of work will differ and therefore making inferences about the effect of load alone may be open to debate. Further, in research studies employing the kettlebell swing, there has seemingly been no standardisation of swing speed or cadence. Modification of swing cadence may result in different intensities of exercise, particularly if swing volume is set as a product of a set duration. The current study seeks to address this issue by comparing the physiological and mechanical responses to kettlebell swings at different loads and swing speeds. We hypothesized that heavier kettlebell load and faster swing speeds would elicit greater physiological and mechanical responses compared to lighter kettlebell load and slower swing speed.

2. Method, Results, Discussion

2.1. Method

2.1.1. Participants

Following institutional ethics approval, briefing regarding the study and provision of written informed consent, 16 strength trained participants (10 males, six females; mean age $\pm$ S.D. = 23 $\pm$ 2.9 years, height = 176.2 $\pm$ 9.2 cm, body mass = 76.3 $\pm$ 14.7 kg) volunteered to participate. Participants were recruited from the pool of MSc Strength and Conditioning Students at the institution where the testing took place. All participants had experience performing resistance exercise, including work with kettlebells, and were free of any musculoskeletal pain or disorders. Inclusion criteria included currently participating in > 10 h week^{-1} programmed physical activity including strength and endurance based activities and prior experience using kettlebells. Exclusion criteria included any musculoskeletal injury that would have prevented engagement in the experimental protocol. Mean $\pm$ S.D. of years training experience was 4.5 $\pm$ 1.5 years.

2.1.2. Procedures

This study used a within groups, repeated measures design, where participants undertook five visits to the human performance laboratory. The first visit was for familiarisation, and the subsequent four visits were counterbalanced experimental trials, which were all performed at the same time of day to minimise circadian variation. Participants were asked to refrain from strenuous exercise in the 24 h before exercise and to attend the laboratory in a hydrated state (e.g., minimum water consumption of 500 mL in the 3 h before testing). Participants engaged in the following four trials: 2 min kettlebell swings with an 8 kg kettlebell at a fast cadence; 2 min kettlebell swings with an 8 kg kettlebell at a slow cadence; 4 min kettlebell swings with a 4 kg kettlebell at a fast cadence; 4 min kettlebell swings with a 4 kg kettlebell at a slow cadence. Heart Rate (HR) and RPE were assessed at mid and end points of each bouts of swings. Blood lactate (BLa) was determined following each swing bout using a 5 µL capillary blood sample taken from the fingertip (Lactate Pro, Arkray Instruments, Kyoto, Japan). Peak net vertical force was also calculated from force platform data (AMTI AccuGait, Watertown, MA, USA), collected throughout each bout of kettlebell swings. Slow and fast cadence was determined via pilot work where different swing speeds were performed by an experienced strength and conditioning professional with 4 and 8 kg kettlebells. From this the two cadences chosen to represent slow (40 BPM) and fast (80 BPM) were selected as being ecologically sound in terms of use within fitness and strength and conditioning programmes. Throughout all trials a metronome (Seiko SQ44, Tokyo, Japan) was used to regulate cadence with a full swing (upwards and downwards phase) being completed in 2 BPM. This resulted in 20 full swings being completed per minute in the slow conditions and 40 full swings being completed in the fast conditions. In this manner, the total work completed in the slow and fast swing speed condition was the same when comparing across 4 kg and 8 kg kettlebell loads. All swings were performed in accordance with the technique reported by Tsatsouline [1] and as used in prior studies examining kettlebell swing performance [8]. Participants were positioned with feet shoulder width apart and standing on the force platform for each trial. Prior to each trial, all participants completed a 5 min warm up protocol at 25 W on a cycle ergometer (Monark, Vansbro, Sweden). They then began each trial 2 min after completion of the warm-up.

2.1.3. Statistical Analysis

In order to examine any changes in Heart Rate, Rating of Perceived Exertion and peak force, a series of 2 (4 kg *vs.* 2 kg kettlebell load) × 2 (slow *vs.* fast swing speed) × 2 (time, mid point *vs.* end point) ways repeated measures analysis of variance (ANOVA) were used. Any differences in post exercise blood lactate were examined using repeated measures ANOVA. Where any statistical differences were found, Bonferroni post-hoc multiple comparisons were used to determine where the differences lay. Partial η^2 ($P\eta^2$) was used as a measure of effect size. The statistical package for social sciences (SPSS, version 22, IBM Inc, New York, NY, USA) was used for all analysis and statistical significance was set as $P = 0.05$ *a priori*.

2.2. Results

In regard to heart rate, results indicated no significant higher order interaction or main effects due to load or cadence (all $P = > 0.05$). However, there was a significant main effect for time ($P = 0.001$, $P\eta^2 = 0.621$), whereby heart rate at mid-point in each trial was significantly lower than heart rate at the end point of each trial ($P = 0.001$). Mean ± SE of heart rate was 148.1 ± 4.1 BPM and 155.5 ± 3.8 BPM at mid and end points respectively. There was also no significant difference in peak Bla across conditions ($P = 0.377$). For RPE there was a significant Load X cadence interaction ($P = 0.030$, $P\eta^2 = 0.293$, see Figure 1) where RPE was higher during the 8 kg slow cadence condition compared to the 4 kg fast cadence and 4 kg slow cadence condition. Post hoc analysis indicated that there was a significant difference between 8 kg load at a slow cadence and 4 kg load at a slow cadence ($P = 0.002$) and 8 kg load at a slow cadence and 4 kg load at a fast cadence ($P = 0.016$). When peak vertical force was examined there were no significant differences between loads, cadence or time points (all $P > 0.05$). Mean ± SE of heart rate, peak blood lactate concentration and peak vertical force across loads and cadences and at mid and end point in each trial are presented in Table 1.

2.3. Discussion

The current study compared physiological, perceptual and mechanical variables during the kettlebell swing at two different loads and two different cadences. This is the first study to date to examine this issue in a manner where total work can be equalised across loads and cadence. The results of this study demonstrate that when this is the case the physiological and mechanical responses are similar between 4 and 8 kg kettlebells. However, when the 8 kg kettlebell swings at a slow cadence produced significantly higher perception of exertion than any of the other conditions. For strength and conditioning coaches and athletes this has useful implications for the development of kettlebell training programmes in that a heavier load (8 kg) when swung more slowly results in higher RPEs when the physiological and mechanical response is the same. In such cases, adherence to training programmes might be more effective if using a 4 kg load on the basis that it will feel more comfortable but elicit the same physiological response as an 8 kg load.

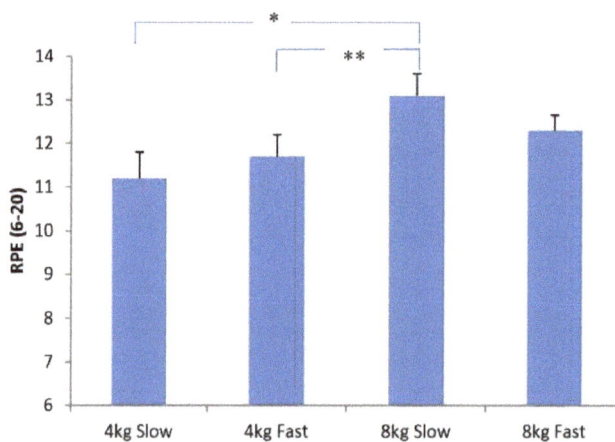

Figure 1. Mean $\pm$ SE of RPE values during kettlebell swings across loads and cadences (* $P = 0.002$, ** $P = 0.016$).

Table 1. Mean (SE) of heart rate, peak blood lactate concentration and peak vertical force at the mid point and end point of kettlebell swings at different loads and cadences.

	4 kg Slow		4 kg Fast		8 kg Slow		8 kg Fast	
	Mid Point	End Point	Mid Point	End Point	Mid Point	End Point	Mid Point	End Point
HR (BPM)	144 (4.8)	151 (4.4)	148 (3.9)	155 (3.7)	148 (7.1)	160 (4.3)	150 (3.7)	155 (4.2)
Bla (mmol/L)	-	5.8 (1.1)	-	4.9 (.55)	-	7.5 (1.6)	-	5.8 (1.1)
Peak Force (N)	562.5 (67.0)	551.2 (63.1)	516.2 (126.3)	462.9 (136.8)	623.1 (60.1)	585.4 (56.3)	557.6 (112.2)	539.3 (112.1)

In some respects it is difficult to compare the results of this study to prior work that has employed kettlebells as previous studies by Thomas *et al.* [7], Hulsey *et al.* [10], Lake and Lauder [10] have used discrete bouts of kettlebell exercise at different loads. Thus, the differences they report may be a consequence of greater work completed rather than a difference in the load employed. The results present in the current study build on this work by also examining different swing cadence. Prior research [7,8,10,12] has not tended to standardise or consider the effect of swing speed/cadence on responses to this type of exercise.

Sports 2015, 3, 202–208

There are some limitations of the current study, due to lack of prior literature relating to optimum swing speed, cadence was determined via pilot study by strength and conditioning professionals. The two swing cadences employed may not however be "optimal" and additional research examining across the spectrum of possible swing speeds might be useful in determining whether there is an "optimum" kettlebell swing speed. Likewise, two relatively light loads (4 kg and 8 kg) were utilised in the present study. This was again based on pilot data in terms of what loads might conceivably be used for kettlebell swing durations over 2 min in duration. Research designs employed by previous authors have used kettlebell loads in excess of those used in the current study, and up to 32 kg e.g., [8]. They have also tended to use much longer durations of kettlebell swinging, which may lack ecological validity. For example, Hulsey *et al.* [10] employed a continuous 10 min period of kettlebell swings and Thomas *et al.* [7] employed three sets of 10 min kettlebell swings, each separated by a 3 min rest period. Such durations of kettlebell exercise seem in excess of what would realistically be engaged in within a gym setting, and particularly physically demanding. Hence the decision in the present to design to employ a smaller duration of swings, more akin to what might be used by the general exercising public. In addition only net peak net vertical force was assessed in the present study and future work that presents an analysis of overall mechanical demands, as well as asymmetry, may elucidate further information in relation to the biomechanics of the kettlebell swing. In regard to practical application, this study suggests that, when matched for work, 4 kg and 8 kg kettlebells when swung at fast or slow cadence, produce similar physiological and mechanical responses but the perceptual response was greater when the kettlebell was swung with an 8 kg load at a slow cadence. Thus, coaches and athletes may likely benefit to the same extent by swinging a 4 kg kettlebell than an 8 kg kettlebell.

3. Conclusion

The present study indicates that the physiological response to kettlebell swings at slow and fast cadences with 4 and 8 kg kettlebells is similar, as is the peak net vertical force. Perceived exertion values are higher when using an 8 kg kettlebell with a slow swing cadence. For coaches and athletes a 4 kg kettlebell swing protocol may be preferable as it results in similar physiological and mechanical response but lower RPE as compared to an 8 kg protocol.

Author Contributions: Michael J. Duncan, Rosanna Gibbard, Leanne M. Raymond and Peter Mundy designed the study, Rosanna Gibbard and Leanne M. Raymond collected the data. Michael J. Duncan and Peter Mundy analysed and interpreted the data. Michael J. Duncan, Rosanna Gibbard, Leanne M. Raymond and Peter Mundy wrote the manuscript. All authors critically reviewed, contributed to and approved the manuscript.

Conflicts of Interest: The authors declare no conflict of interest

References

1. Tsatsouline, P. *Enter the Kettlebell*; Dragon Door Publications: St. Paul, MN, USA, 2006.
2. O'Hara, R.B.; Serres, J.; Traver, K.L.; Wright, B.; Vojta, C.; Eveland, E. The influence of non-traditional training modalities in physical performance: Review of the Literature. *Aviat Space Environ. Med.* **2012**, *83*, 985–990. [CrossRef] [PubMed]
3. Brumitt, J.; En Gilpin, H.; Brunette, M.; Meira, E.P. Incorporating kettlebells into a lower extremity sports rehabilitation program. *North Am. J. Sports Phys. Ther.* **2010**, *5*, 257–265.
4. Zebis, M.K.; Skotte, J.; Andersen, C.H.; Mortensen, P.; Petersen, M.H.; Viskaer, T.C.; Jensen, T.L.; Bencke, J.; Andersen, L.L. Kettlebell swing targets semitendinosus and supine leg curl targets biceps femoris: An EMG study with rehabilitation implications. *Br. J. Sports Med.* **2013**, *47*, 1192–1198. [CrossRef] [PubMed]
5. Jay, K.; Frisch, D.; Hansen, K.; Zebis, M.K.; Andersen, C.H.; Mortensen, O.S.; Andersen, L.L. Kettlebell training for musculoskeletal and cardiovascular health: A randomized controlled trial. *Scand. J. Work Environ. Health* **2011**, *37*, 196–203. [CrossRef] [PubMed]
6. Farrar, R.E.; Mayhew, J.L.; Koch, A.J. Oxygen cost of kettlebell swings. *J. Strength Cond. Res.* **2010**, *24*, 1034–1036. [CrossRef] [PubMed]

Sports **2015**, *3*, 202–208

7. Thomas, J.F.; Larson, K.L.; Hollander, D.B.; Kraemer, R.R. Comparison of two-hand kettlebell exercise and graded treadmill walking: Effectiveness as a stimulus for cardiorespiratory fitness. *J. Strength Cond. Res.* **2014**, *28*, 998–1006. [CrossRef] [PubMed]

8. Lake, J.P.; Lauder, M.A. Mechanical demands of kettlebell swing exercise. *J. Strength Cond. Res.* **2012**, *26*, 3209–3216. [CrossRef] [PubMed]

9. McGill, S.M.; Marshall, L.W. Kettlebell swing, snatch, and bottoms-up carry: Back and hip muscle activation, motion, and low back loads. *J. Strength Cond. Res.* **2012**, *26*, 16–27. [CrossRef] [PubMed]

10. Husley, C.R.; Soto, D.T.; Koch, A.J.; Mayhew, J.L. Comparison of kettlebell swings and treadmill running at equivalent RPE Values. *J. Strength Cond. Res.* **2012**, *26*, 1203–1207.

11. Beardsley, C.; Contreras, B. The role of kettlebells in strength and conditioning: A review of the Literature. *Strength Cond. J.* **2014**, *36*, 64–70. [CrossRef]

12. Borg, G. Perceived exertion as an indicator of somatic stress. *Scand. J. Rehab. Med.* **1970**, *2*, 92–98.

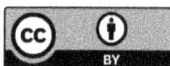

sports

MDPI

Article

A Comparison of Upper Body Strength between Rock Climbing and Resistance Trained Men

Kristina M. Macias [†], Lee E. Brown [†,*], Jared W. Coburn [†] and David D. Chen [†]

Human Performance Laboratory, Department of Kinesiology, California State University, Fullerton, 800 N State College Blvd, Fullerton, CA 92831, USA; Kristina.macias@gmail.com (K.M.M.); jcoburn@fullerton.edu (J.W.C.); dapchen@fullerton.edu (D.D.C.)
* Correspondence: leebrown@fullerton.edu; Tel.: +1-657-278-4605; Fax: +1-657-278-1366
† These authors contributed equally to this work.

Academic Editor: Eling de Bruin
Received: 3 July 2015; Accepted: 28 July 2015; Published: 30 July 2015

Abstract: Studies have shown that advanced rock climbers have greater upper body strength than that of novice climbers or non-climbers. The purpose of this study was to compare upper body strength between rock climbing and resistance trained men. Fifteen resistance trained men (age 25.28 ± 2.26 yrs; height 177.45 ± 4.08 cm; mass 85.17 ± 10.23 kg; body fat $10.13 \pm 5.40\%$) and 15 rock climbing men (age 23.25 ± 2.23 yrs; height 175.57 ± 8.03 cm; mass 66.66 ± 9.40 kg; body fat $6.86 \pm 3.82\%$) volunteered to participate. Rock climbing (RC) men had been climbing for at least two years, 2–3 times a week, able to climb at least a boulder rating of V4–5 and had no current injuries. Resistance trained (RT) men had been total body strength training for at least two years, 2–3 times a week with no current injuries. Each participant performed pull-ups to failure, grip strength, and pinch strength. RT were significantly older and heavier than RC. RC performed significantly more pull-ups (19.31 ± 4.31) than RT (15.64 ± 4.82). RC had greater relative pinch strength (R 0.27 ± 0.10 kg/kg; L 0.24 ± 0.07 kg/kg) than RT (R 0.19 ± 0.04 kg/kg; L 0.16 ± 0.05 kg/kg) and greater relative grip strength (R 0.70 ± 0.10 kg/kg; L 0.65 ± 0.12 kg/kg) than RT (R 0.57 ± 0.14 kg/kg; L 0.56 ± 0.15 kg/kg). Overall, RC men demonstrated greater performance in tests involving relative strength when compared to RT men. Rock climbing can promote increased upper body strength even in the absence of traditional resistance training.

Keywords: grip; finger; pinch; pull-ups; push-ups; relative

1. Introduction

Rock climbing involves lifting their body mass by pulling with their upper body musculature and using many different handholds and grips, including a wide 4-finger pinch and a small two finger pinch. This requires significant finger, grip and upper body strength. Balas [1] demonstrated that a higher climbing volume and an eight week training program resulted in increased grip and relative upper body strength of youth climbers. They also observed that hand-arm strength and endurance, body composition and climbing volume combined were predictors of climbing performance. Studies have also shown a significant difference in grip and pinch maximal voluntary contraction (MVC) in elite climbers when compared to recreational and non-climbers [2–6].

Predictors of climbing ability include upper body strength, grip and finger strength, along with high relative strength and lower body fat [7,8]. Elite climbers exhibit significantly greater strength than recreational climbers and non-climbers and this is seen even more prominent when the grip is more climbing specific [5,6,9]. Limonta *et al.* [2] observed a higher maximal voluntary contraction and a significant difference in endurance time between elite climbers and sedentary individuals during controlled fatiguing contractions in finger flexor muscles. Grant [4] determined that elite climbers had significantly greater flexibility (leg span), upper body strength (pull-ups and bent arm hang), and left and right pincer strength than recreational climbers and physically active non-climbers.

Based on the previous studies, rock climbing appears to have an important upper body strength component, which is derived from that training. Studies have observed significant differences in handgrip and pincer strength between climbers and sedentary individuals [3,4]. However, there is a paucity of research comparing strength of those involved in high-level rock climbing and traditional resistance training. Therefore, the purpose of this study was to compare upper body strength between rock climbers and resistance-trained men. We hypothesized that resistance trained men would exhibit significantly greater absolute grip due to their traditional training. Another hypothesis was that climbers would exhibit superior relative strength due to their experience with bodyweight support activity.

2. Materials and Methods

2.1. Participants

All participants were males between the ages of 20–29 with no injuries in the past six months that would prevent them from completing each task. Climbers had at least two years' experience, climbed indoors 2–3 times per week, outdoors at least once a month and did not participate in a structured resistance training program. Each participant was considered a self-reported "advanced" climber with at least a Hueco Scale rating of V4–5 (on a V0–16 scale) [10]. Resistance-trained men had at least two years' experience in full body lifting consisting of squats, deadlift, bench press and pull-ups. At the beginning of each visit, subjects signed a university IRB approved informed consent document. Then height and weight were recorded on a stadiometer (216, Seca Corporation, Ontario, CA, USA) and weight scale (ES200L, Ohaus Corporation, Pinebrook, NJ, USA).

2.2. Body Fat Percentage

Skinfold thickness was measured to the nearest .5mm using skinfold calipers (Lange, Santa Cruz, CA, USA). Two measurements were taken on the right side of the body (chest, abdomen and thigh) and the average of the values was recorded for analysis. Body fat percentage was estimated using the Jackson and Pollock equation [11].

2.3. Pull-Ups

For all performance tests, subjects performed at least three repetitions for warm-up and familiarization until they could execute the test per the specific guidelines, then rested for 2 min. Pull-ups and push-ups were counterbalanced. They completed the maximum number of pronated pull-ups possible in one minute [12]. They were positioned hanging from the bar with arms at full extension then pulled up so their chin reached the top of the bar then lowered themselves back down to full arm extension with their legs also fully extended [4]. If they used any momentum from their lower body as assistance the repetition was not counted. They were able to rest with arms at full extension, but if they let go of the bar the test was terminated.

2.4. Push-Ups

They laid prone on the floor and placed their thumbs at shoulder width, kept their body in a straight line and touched their chin to a tennis ball at the bottom of each repetition [13]. A cadence was set to 80 beats per minute (40 push-ups per minute) with a metronome and the test lasted a maximum of two min. When they were unable to keep the cadence or stopped due to fatigue, the test was terminated. [14].

2.5. Finger Strength

Participants rested for 5 min before finger strength tests were administered. A Flexiforce sensor (Model A201, South Boston, MA, USA) was used to measure finger strength between the thumb and all four fingers (1 = index, 2 = middle, 3 = ring, and 4 = little finger) [15]. They squeezed putty grip (Power putty) five times with each hand for warm-up, then rested 2 min. They were seated in an upright position with their arm placed on a table that was adjusted so that the elbow and shoulder joints were flexed to 90 degrees. Starting with the thumb and index finger, they placed the finger lightly over the sensor with the thumb opposed. The other fingers were curled under to prevent them from assisting when the sensor was squeezed. When signaled, they gradually squeezed the sensor for 5 s leading to maximal force. Next the thumb and middle finger were tested, with only the ring and little finger curled under. Then the ring finger was tested with only the little finger curled under. Finally, the little finger was tested last. Each finger on each hand was measured alternately three times with 15 s rest and the best of the three repetitions was recorded for analysis. Relative values were determined by dividing strength by body mass (kg/kg).

2.6. Pinch Strength

A handgrip dynamometer (T.K.K5401 Takei Koyo, Tokyo, Japan) was used to measure pinch strength. Participants squeezed putty grip (Power putty) five times with each hand for warm-up, then rested 2 min. The dynamometer was set to 4.5 cm wide [4]. They were seated in an upright position exactly the same as for finger strength with the dynamometer digital display facing away. They grasped the moveable arm of the dynamometer with four fingertips and the thumb opposed and braced around the immovable part of the device, while the administrator held the device stable [16]. Measurements were taken alternately between left and right hands with 15 s rest. Each hand was measured three times and the best of the three repetitions was recorded for analysis. Relative values were determined by dividing strength by body mass (kg/kg).

2.7. Grip Strength

The same handgrip dynamometer was used for measurement. The size of the grip was adjusted so that the second joint of the middle finger was positioned at 90 degrees. Participants were seated in an upright position on a box that was 47 cm tall, while holding the dynamometer in one hand, arm at their side with the digital display facing away. They squeezed the dynamometer for 5 s leading to maximal force then released [17]. Measurements were taken alternately between the left and right hands with 15 s rest. Each hand was measured three times and the best of the three repetitions was recorded for analysis. Relative values were determined by dividing strength by body mass (kg/kg).

2.8. Statistical Analyses

Two independent t-tests analyzed pull-ups and push-ups between groups. Multiple 2×2 (group $\times$ hand) mixed factor ANOVAs analyzed absolute and relative grip and absolute and relative pinch strength. Multiple $2 \times 2 \times 4$ (group $\times$ hand $\times$ finger) mixed factor ANOVAs analyzed absolute and relative finger strength. Main effects were followed up with *t*-tests or LSD post hoc tests. Alpha level was set a-priori at 0.05.

3. Results

RT were significantly older and heavier than RC, but height and body fat percentage were not significantly different (Table 1).

Table 1. Mean ± SD of age, height, mass and body composition between resistance trained (RT) and rock climbing (RC) men.

Variable	RT	RC
Age (yrs)	25.28 ± 2.26*	23.25 ± 2.23
Height (cm)	177.45 ± 4.08	175.57 ± 8.03
Mass (kg)	85.17 ± 10.23*	66.66 ± 9.40
Body Fat (%)	10.13 ± 5.40	6.86 ± 3.82

Note: * Significantly (age $P = 0.02$; mass $P = 0.02$) greater than RC.

For pull-ups and push-ups, RC performed a significantly greater number of pull-ups than RT, but push-ups were not significantly different (Table 2).

Table 2. Mean ± SD of pull-ups and push-ups between resistance trained (RT) and rock climbing (RC) men.

Performance	RT	RC
Pull-ups (#)	15.64 ± 4.82	19.31 ± 4.31*
Push-ups (#)	38.28 ± 4.89	34.56 ± 8.13

Note: * Significantly ($P = 0.03$) greater than RT.

For absolute grip, there was no interaction or main effect for group but there was a main effect for hand with the right being stronger than the left. For relative grip, there was no interaction but there was a main effect for hand with the right being stronger than the left and a main effect for group with RC having significantly greater relative grip strength than RT (Table 3).

Table 3. Mean ± SD of left and right absolute and relative grip between resistance trained (RT) and rock climbing (RC) men and combined total for both groups.

Performance	RT	RC	Group Total
R grip (kg)	49.26 ± 14.16	46.15 ± 6.24	47.60 ± 10.61#
L grip (kg)	48.45 ± 15.42	43.16 ± 6.33	45.63 ± 11.60
R gripREL (kg/kg)	0.57 ± 0.14	0.70 ± 0.10	0.64 ± 0.14#
L gripREL (kg/kg)	0.56 ± 0.15	0.65 ± 0.12	0.61 ± 0.14
R&Lavg gripREL (kg/kg)	0.56 ± 0.14	0.67 ± 0.11*	-

Note: # Significantly (absolute $P = 0.03$; relative $P = 0.01$) greater than left; * Significantly ($P = 0.02$) greater than RT.

For absolute pinch, there was no interaction or main effect for group but there was a main effect for hand with the right being stronger than the left. For relative pinch, there was no interaction but there were main effects for group and hand. RC had significantly greater relative pinch strength than RT (Table 4).

Table 4. Mean ± SD of left and right absolute and relative pinch strength between resistance trained (RT) and rock climbing (RC) men and combined total for both groups.

Performance	RT	RC	Group Total
R pinch (kg)	16.07 ± 3.00	18.03 ± 7.01	17.11 ± 5.52#
L pinch (kg)	14.15 ± 4.65	16.11 ± 5.35	15.19 ± 5.05
R pinchREL (kg/kg)	0.19 ± 0.04	0.27 ± 0.10	0.23 ± 0.08#
L pinchREL (kg/kg)	0.16 ± 0.05	0.24 ± 0.07	0.20 ± 0.07
R&Lavg pinchREL (kg/kg)	0.18 ± 0.04	0.25 ± 0.08*	-

Note: # Significantly (absolute $P = 0.00$; relative $P = 0.00$) greater than left; * Significantly ($P = 0.00$) greater than RT.

For absolute and relative finger strength there were no significant three way or two-way interactions or main effects for group or hand. However, there was a main effect for fingers for both. Both absolute (Figure 1) and relative (Figure 2) finger strength were followed up with LSD post hoc tests for pairwise comparisons that showed the first finger was significantly stronger than fingers three and four. The second finger was significantly stronger than fingers one, three and four. The third finger was significantly stronger than finger four.

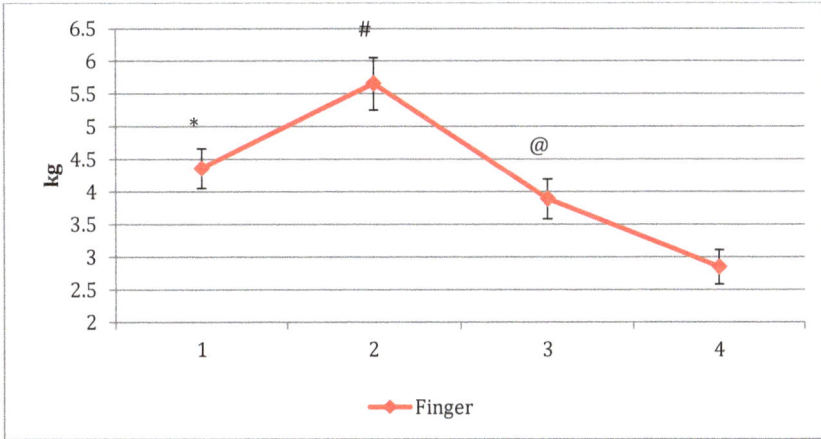

Figure 1. Mean ± SD of absolute finger strength. 1 = index, 2 = middle. 3 = ring and 4 = little. * Significantly (*P* = 0.00) greater than fingers 3 and 4; # Significantly (*P* = 0.00) greater than fingers 1,3 and 4; @ Significantly (*P* = 0.00) greater than finger 4.

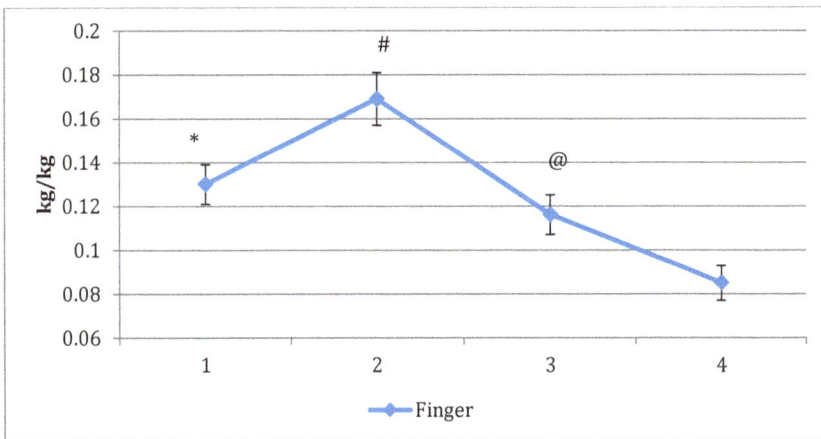

Figure 2. Mean ± SD of relative finger strength. 1 = index, 2 = middle. 3 = ring and 4 = little. * Significantly (*P* = 0.00) greater than fingers 3 and 4; # Significantly (*P* = 0.00) greater than fingers 1,3 and 4; @ Significantly (*P* = 0.00) greater than finger 4.

4. Discussion

The purpose of this study was to compare upper body strength between rock climbing and resistance trained men. The main findings were that rock climbers performed a significantly (*P* = 0.03) greater number of pull-ups, and had significantly greater relative grip ($P = 0.01$) and relative pinch ($P = 0.00$) strength than resistance trained men. This may be due to the physical demands required of rock climbing men to negotiate challenging routes successfully. These demands include lifting their body mass by pulling with their upper body musculature and supporting their body weight by many different handholds and grips [7,8]. Requirements for these demands include low body mass, strong pulling, pinching, and gripping strength to support body weight movements, and a large climbing volume in order to see increased relative strength and climbing ability [4,9,17]. In contrast, resistance trained men perform traditional weight room exercises and generally demonstrate greater absolute upper body strength but less relative strength than climbers. Grip strength of resistance trained men is developed through upper, and lower body exercises [18,19]. Climbers strengthen their upper body by lifting their own body mass and by directly working the grip via pinching and gripping [1,4,17]. Resistance trained men utilize exercises that indirectly strengthen their grip (*i.e.*, push-ups, squats, leg press, *etc.*) [18,19]. Therefore, it appears that both activities may be utilized to improve upper body strength.

In this study, we found that although groups were similar in height, climbers had significantly less body mass when compared to resistance trained men. This is probably due to the specific demands of each respective activity. Schweizer [20] determined that climbers had low levels of body mass and that body weight and height were negatively correlated with climbing performance. The current study corroborates that climbers' lower body mass probably led to greater relative strength.

In a contrasting study, Grant [4] demonstrated that there were no significant differences between elite, recreational and non-climbers for body mass, height, height:body mass ratio, or body fat %. It is important to note that they compared climbers to other climbers, not resistance trained men. So it is not known whether the elite climbers would have been significantly different in mass and body fat when compared to the resistance trained men of the current study. It is clear that low body fat and mass are desirable to climbers, however, there are numerous other variables that are used to determine climbing level such as type of training, climbing volume, grip, pinch, and finger strength [1,4,9,17]. For resistance trained men, training leads to hypertrophy and increased body mass which results in greater strength. This may be why resistance trained men in our study had significantly greater body mass. Despite differences in training, each group's goals overlap to some degree. Both desire increased upper body strength, which improves grip strength.

Balas [1] concluded that the practice of rock climbing resulted in increased upper body strength. He had young climbers, with little or no experience, participate in an 8-week climbing program and saw a significant increase in upper body strength, specifically, relative grip strength. In a similar study [17], he demonstrated that climbing volume and experience can predict performance, with a notable relationship between number of meters climbed per week, body fat, grip and bent-arm hang. Our results correspondingly showed that rock climbers had significantly greater relative pinch and grip strength. These two different grip types were chosen to be tested for the purpose of variation and specificity. The pinch is more climbing specific and the grip is more resistance training specific. It seems reasonable that if climbers utilized resistance training, focusing on larger lifts, it would result in improved upper body strength. However, a significant increase in mass might decrease climbing performance.

Several studies have shown that elite or advanced climbers demonstrate significantly greater MVC in a grip or pinch test [4,9,17,21]. Green [21] saw that trained climbers (similar to those in this study) had a significantly greater MVC and intermittent exercise capacity than untrained climbers. The conclusion is that climbing directly increases grip strength, similar to the current study.

Resistance training is commonly used to increase upper body strength. Thomas [18] observed the effects of a resistance training program on handgrip strength in young adults. Their results indicated that even though none of the movements in the training program involved specifically strengthening grip, each exercise contributed to overall improvement of absolute grip strength of the right hand only. Another study by Wilmore [19] supports resistance training as a way to improve handgrip strength. Subjects participated in a training program that consisted of basic strength exercises and increased their absolute grip strength even though none of the exercises specifically strengthened handgrip. We hypothesized in the current study that resistance trained men would exhibit significantly greater absolute grip strength because absolute strength is the primary outcome of resistance training. However, we observed no difference between groups but climbers had significantly greater relative grip and pinch strength. Once again, this is probably due to climbers having less body mass.

Another hypothesis was that climbers would exhibit superior performance in tests of relative strength, such as push-ups and pull-ups. This was partially confirmed as climbers performed significantly more pull-ups than resistance trained men. Again, probably a result of climbers having significantly less body mass. Additionally, pull-ups are a very common movement performed in climbing and could lead to greater muscular endurance in rock climbers. Grant [4] also observed that elite climbers were able to perform significantly more pull-ups than recreational and non-climbers. In contrast, push-ups demonstrated no significant difference between groups. Push-ups were one of the exercises Balas [1] utilized in the resistance training program that indirectly improved grip strength. This suggests that push-ups could be part of a rock climbers training routine to aid in strengthening the upper body while also working the anterior chain in addition to the posterior chain, which is most often utilized while climbing. Resistance trained men are also at a slight disadvantage during push-ups as they must support greater overall body mass [13].

We did not find a significant difference in finger strength between groups. In contrast, Grant [4] found a significant difference in finger strength between elite and recreational climbers, but only for a climbing specific grip. The sensor used in the current study was very thin, making it less specific to a climbing grip and may not be a valid indicator of climbing finger strength. In addition, the resistance trained men were not familiar with the finger strength position.

Finally, Grant [9] compared climbing specific finger endurance in intermediate rock climbers, rowers, and aerobically trained men. This is the most similar study to ours comparing rock climbers to resistance trained men. Since the rowers followed a resistance training program it was thought that they would perform similarly to climbers. However, climbers demonstrated significantly greater MVC of a climbing specific grip when compared to rowers and aerobically trained men, but there was no difference between groups in endurance. These results further support that climbing directly improves grip strength.

5. Conclusions

Climbers demonstrated significantly greater relative grip and pinch strength and were also able to perform significantly more pull-ups than resistance trained men, due to their significantly lower body mass. Therefore, training for rock climbing should promote increased upper body strength in the absence of increased mass as relative strength appears to be an important parameter in this population. Additionally, testing rock climbers should focus on relative upper body strength as a positive indicator of performance.

Author Contributions: Kristina Macias, Lee Brown, Jared Coburn and David Chen were involved in study design, data collection, data interpretation, and manuscript writing.

Conflicts of Interest: The authors declare no conflict of interest.

References

1. Balas, J.; Strejcova, B.; Maly, T.; Mala, L.; Martin, A.J. Changes in upper body strength and body composition after 8 weeks indoor climbing in youth. *Isok. Exer. Sci.* **2009**, *17*, 173–179.
2. Limonta, E.; Ce, E.; Veicsteinas, A.; Esposito, F. Force control during fatiguing contractions in elite rock climbers. *Sport Sci. Health.* **2008**, *4*, 37–42. [CrossRef]
3. Fanchini, M.; Violette, F.; Impellizzerim, F.M.; Maffiuletti, N.A. Differences in climbing-specific strength between boulder and lead rock climbers. *J. Strength Cond. Res.* **2013**, *27*, 310–314. [CrossRef] [PubMed]

4. Grant, S.; Hynes, V.; Whittaker, A.; Aitchison, T. Anthropometric, strength, endurance, flexibility characteristics of elite and recreational climbers. *J. Sport Sci.* **1996**, *14*, 301–309. [CrossRef] [PubMed]
5. Grant, S.; Hasler, T.; Dvies, C.; Aitchison, T.C.; Wilson, J.; Whittaker, A. A comparison of anthropometric, strength, endurance and flexibility characteristics of female elite and recreational climbers and non-climbers. *J. Sport Sci.* **2001**, *19*, 499–505. [CrossRef] [PubMed]
6. MacLeod, D.; Sutherland, D.L.; Buntin, L.; Whitaker, A.; Aitchison, T.; Watt, I.; Bradley, J.; Grant, S. Physiological determinants of climbing-specific finger endurance and sport rock climbing performance. *J. Sports Sci.* **2006**, *25*, 1433–1443. [CrossRef] [PubMed]
7. Schweizer, A.; Schneider, A.; Geohner, K. Dynamic eccentric-concentric strength training of the finger flexors to improve rock-climbing performance. *Isok. Exer. Sci.* **2007**, *15*, 131–136.
8. Mermier, C.M.; Janot, J.M.; Parker, D.L.; Swan, J.G. Physiological and anthropometric determinants of sport climbing performance. *Brit. J. Sports Med.* **2000**, *34*, 359–366. [CrossRef]
9. Grant, S.; Shields, C.; Fitzpatrick, V.; Ming Loh, W.; Whitaker, A.; Watt, I.; Kay, J.W. Climbing-specific finger endurance: A comparative study of intermediate rock climbers, rowers, and aerobically trained individuals. *J. Sports Sci.* **2003**, *21*, 621–630. [CrossRef] [PubMed]
10. Simon, B.; Draper, N.; Hodgson, C.; Blackwell, G. Development of a performance assessment tool for rock climbers. *Eur. J. Sport Sci.* **2009**, *9*, 159–167.
11. Jackson, A.S.; Pollock, M.L. Generalized equations for predicting body density of men. *Br. J. Nutr.* **1978**, *40*, 497–504. [CrossRef] [PubMed]
12. Chen, K.W.; Chiu, P.K.; Lin, I.; Xu, K.F.; Hsu, M.; Liang, M.T. Study of basic military training of the physical fitness and physical self-concept for cadets. *J. Phys. Ed. Rec.* **2007**, *13*, 6–12.
13. Invergo, J.J.; Ball, T.E.; Looney, M. Relationship of push-ups and absolute muscular endurance to bench press strength. *J. Appl. Sport Sci. Res.* **1991**, *5*, 121–125.
14. Plowman, S.A. *Fitnessgram/Activitygram Reference Guide*, 4th ed.; Plowman, S.A., Meredith, M.D., Eds.; The Cooper Institute: Dallas, TX, USA, 2013.
15. Lee, S.; Kong, Y.; Lowe, B.; Song, S. Handle grip span for optimizing finger-specific force capability as a function of hand size. *Ergonomics* **2009**, *52*, 601–608. [CrossRef] [PubMed]
16. Bacon, N.T.; Wingo, J.E.; Richardson, M.T.; Ryan, G.A.; Pangallo, T.C.; Bishop, P.A. Effect of two recovery methods on repeated closed-handed and open-handed weight assisted pull-ups. *J. Strength Cond. Res.* **2012**, *26*, 1348–1352. [CrossRef] [PubMed]
17. Balas, J.; Pecha, O.; Martin, A.J.; Cochrane, D. Hand-arm strength and endurance as predictors of climbing performance. *Europ. J. Sport Sci.* **2011**, *12*, 16–25. [CrossRef]
18. Thomas, E.M.; Shalber, M.; Svantesson, U. The effect of resistance training on handgrip strength and young adults. *Isok. Exer. Sci.* **2008**, *16*, 125–131.
19. Wilmore, J.H. Alterations in strength, body composition and anthropometric measurements consequent to a 10-week weight-training program. *Med. Sci. Sports Exer.* **1974**, *1*, 133–138. [CrossRef]
20. Schweizer, A.; Furrer, M. Correlation of forearm strength and sport climbing performance. *Isok. Exer. Sci.* **2007**, *15*, 211–216.
21. Green, J.; Stannard, S. Active recovery strategies and handgrip performance in trained *vs.* untrained climbers. *J. Strength Cond. Res.* **2010**, *24*, 494–501. [CrossRef] [PubMed]

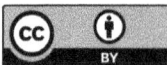

sports

MDPI

Review

Less Is More: The Physiological Basis for Tapering in Endurance, Strength, and Power Athletes

Kevin A. Murach [1,2,*] and James R. Bagley [2]

[1] Department of Rehabilitation Sciences, College of Health Sciences and Center for Muscle Biology, University of Kentucky, MS-508 Chandler Medical Center, 800 Rose Street, Lexington, KY 40508, USA

[2] Department of Kinesiology, College of Health and Social Sciences, San Francisco State University, 1600 Holloway Avenue-Gym 101, San Francisco, CA 94132, USA; jrbagley@sfsu.edu

* Correspondence: kmu236@g.uky.edu; Tel.: +1-859-257-2375

Academic Editor: Lee E. Brown
Received: 10 July 2015; Accepted: 17 August 2015; Published: 21 August 2015

Abstract: Taper, or reduced-volume training, improves competition performance across a broad spectrum of exercise modes and populations. This article aims to highlight the physiological mechanisms, namely in skeletal muscle, by which taper improves performance and provide a practical literature-based rationale for implementing taper in varied athletic disciplines. Special attention will be paid to strength- and power-oriented athletes as taper is under-studied and often overlooked in these populations. Tapering can best be summarized by the adage "less is more" because maintained intensity and reduced volume prior to competition yields significant performance benefits.

Keywords: taper; reduced-volume training; periodization; skeletal muscle; fiber type

1. Introduction

Taper can be defined as a structured reduction in training volume (as compared to peak training load) for a specific period of time prior to athletic competition as a means to enhance performance. In simpler terms, taper is formalized recovery training that occurs after a heavy training block. Rest as an integral aspect of training is not a recent concept. The importance of obligatory recovery time during training was recognized as early as the ancient Olympic games [1]. However, the role of adequate rest in optimizing performance has been more widely publicized in the last 60 years with the concept of periodization [2,3], or varied training (*i.e.*, mode, time, intensity) for a specific goal.

Endurance athletes have systematically practiced relative rest via reduced-volume training as a means to improve performance for at least 50 years. However, Costill and colleagues [4] in 1985 were the first to experimentally evaluate the physiological effects of a specific tapering protocol using competitive swimmers. Since that time, taper's efficacy has been well documented in swimming, cycling, running, triathlon, rowing, strength training, and team sports to name a few. The effects of tapering are apparent from the whole body (macro) [4] to the cell and gene (micro) [5,6] levels and even include psychological improvements [7]. Despite the multitude of data supporting taper's effectiveness, some athletes and coaches still fail to acknowledge its importance and implement the practice. The purpose of this article is to highlight how taper is experimentally shown to enhance athletic performance across multiple exercise modes and populations. An overview of tapering in endurance-type athletes will be provided, but special attention will be paid to strength- and power-oriented athletes for whom tapering is generally less emphasized. Additionally, the discussion will highlight taper-mediated skeletal muscle improvements and provide broad literature-based guidance for tapering. We hope to underscore the necessity for coaches and athletes to employ well-controlled taper regimens during their training programs.

2. How to Taper

An effective taper regimen can be conducted in numerous ways. The duration and type of taper generally varies by sport but the common theme among endurance tapering protocols is a substantial reduction in training volume prior to competition. The literature suggests that an effective taper could be as short as four days [8] and involve reductions in training volume of up to 90% [9,10]. An improperly conducted taper where endurance exercise volume is only reduced by 25% and high- intensity work is increased to compensate will not yield favorable results [11]. Increasing training volume instead of tapering affords no benefits and may hinder performance [12,13]. For most endurance-oriented activities, a taper lasting two to three weeks characterized by a 40%–70% reduction in volume from peak training with maintained intensity will produce significant performance benefits. For a more in-depth review of specific endurance tapering protocols, refer to Mujika *et al.* [14], Bosquet *et al.* [15], and Wilson *et al.* [16].

The nature of taper is less defined in the literature regarding intermittent type athletic disciplines such as strength-focused weightlifting, power-focused Olympic-style weightlifting, and track and field or team sports where both strength and power are emphasized. However, a recent review on tapering in strength sports suggests (similar to endurance athletics) that performance is improved with a 30%–70% reduction in volume (via reduced intra-session volume or less overall training frequency) for up to four weeks with maintained or slightly increased intensity [17]. The tapering literature specific to power athletes is particularly limited. However, a recent investigation found a 25%–40% reduction in resistance training volume (sessions per week) with maintained intensity improved throwing performance after two weeks in track and field athletes [18]. Another study found enhanced maximal power output with a three week taper characterized by a ~75% resistance-training volume reduction, a slight increase in intensity, and maintained sport-specific training in elite rugby players [19]. Similar to endurance athletes, reduced volume with maintained or slightly increased intensity appears to be the key elements for tapering in strength- and power-focused athletes.

3. Magnitude of Performance Benefits with Taper

A properly conducted taper improves race performance across a broad spectrum of athletic activities and populations (Figure 1). It enhances performance in shorter race events (*i.e.*, 50 meter swim, <10 km cycling time trial [TT], 2000 m row) [4,7,13,20–22] as well as middle distance swimming, biking, and running competition [4,5,9,13,20,22–24]. Taper also improves performance indices in longer-duration events such as the duathlon [25], 40 km cycling TT [26], and triathlon [27,28]. For any distance event, it is reasonable to expect that taper will increase performance on the order of 2%–3%. This is no small change when considering that a 3% improvement in a collegiate 8 kilometer runner's performance could account for a 50 s faster race time [5]. Moreover, meaningful performance benefits are not exclusive to endurance and race events with tapering. A 2%–3% improvement in the bench press and squat in strength athletes [29] and a 5%–6% increase in throwing distance can occur in competitive track and field athletes following a taper period [18].

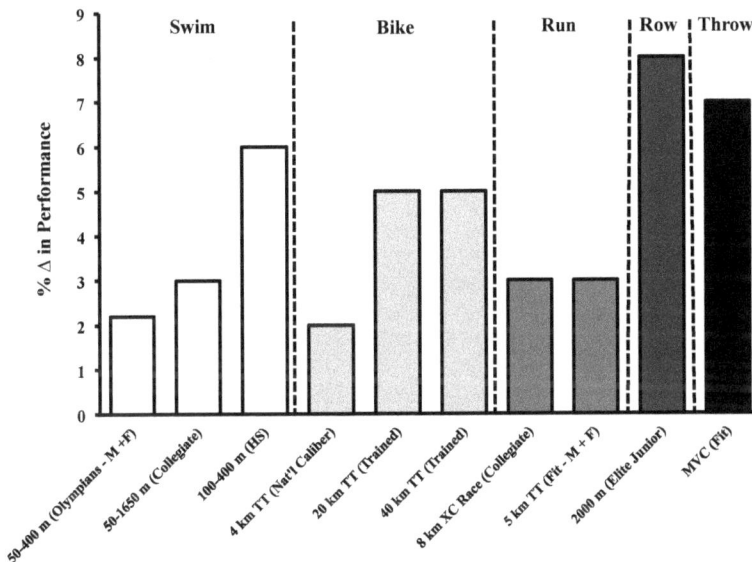

Figure 1. Reported performance benefits from taper in different athletic events and populations. Data were derived from the following studies in order from left to right: Swim-Mujika *et al.* 2002 [30], Costill *et al.* 1985 [4], D'Acquisto *et al.* 1992 [9]. Bike-Berger *et al.* 1999 [7], Neary *et al.* 2003 [24], Neary *et al.* 2003 [26]. Run-Luden *et al.* 2010 [5], Houmard *et al.* 1994 [23]. Row-Steinacker *et al.* 2000 [21]. Throw-Zaras *et al.* 2014 [18]. m = Meter; M = Male; F = Female; HS = High School; TT = Time Trial; T + F = Track and Field.

4. Fitness Is Not Lost with Taper

A common misconception among athletes and coaches is that less training always equates to a loss of fitness. However, the literature indicates that fitness in endurance athletes (measured as aerobic capacity, or VO_{2max}) is not lost following the taper period and five studies have actually shown an increase in fitness with less training [18,21–23,25]. Reducing training volume for as long as four weeks [7] by >85% (in the last week) [6,19] still yields gains in performance without a loss of fitness. Considering the robust adaptations observed with short-duration high-intensity interval training, even in already highly trained individuals [26,27], it should come as no surprise that a well-designed taper of reduced volume and quality high intensity work can preserve fitness for up to a month. In strength athletes, short-term complete rest (≤ 1 week) does not reduce force-producing capacity while tapering only seems to improve strength [17]. To our knowledge, there is little to no evidence in the literature showing that a properly conducted taper does not improve fitness indices in endurance, strength, power, or team sport athletes.

5. Taper and Muscle Energy Usage

If an athlete consistently trains rigorously and with high volumes, one could expect muscle energy stores (*i.e.*, carbohydrate, or glycogen) to be chronically lowered. Logically, a reduction in training volume during taper with proper diet reverses this condition (Figure 2) [10,24]. Initial muscle glycogen levels do not seem to affect short-term high-intensity performance (*i.e.*, a sprint) [31,32]. Indeed, the performance decrements from overtraining [33] and the performance benefits from taper [26] can occur independent of muscle glycogen levels during shorter duration activities. However, initial glycogen levels do affect performance during repeated high-intensity efforts [34,35] as well as endurance efforts lasting ~60 min or more [36,37]. Expanded muscle glycogen stores may therefore be a desirable taper-induced adaptation for endurance athletes, team sport athletes, and during activities requiring multiple individual efforts in quick succession. Other measures related to muscle energy usage such as lactate [4,9,10,13,23,38,39] and aerobic enzymes [8,10,26] are less affected by tapering. Taper-mediated muscle glycogen replenishment enhances performance in some circumstances but does not fully account for the beneficial effects of tapering.

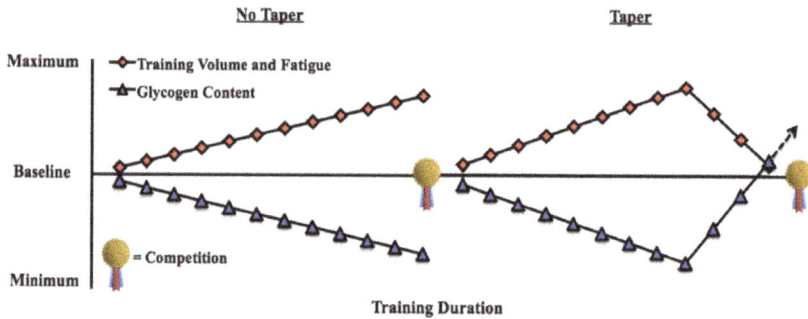

Figure 2. Illustration of training volume, accumulated fatigue, and skeletal muscle glycogen content in response to training with and without taper (assuming proper diet). Concept derived from Sherman *et al.* [37] and Halson *et al.* [40].

6. Taper Improves Muscle Power in Endurance Athletes

Numerous studies spanning various exercise modes and subject populations [21,41–43] have since corroborated the original findings [4] of increased muscle power with taper in endurance athletes (Figure 3). Taper-derived muscle power gains may occur in two phases (early and late) which reinforces that a taper should be of adequate length (generally ≥2 weeks) [43]. One might predict the main effect of tapering in endurance athlete's muscle would be targeted to the highly aerobic slow-twitch muscle fibers. However, it is the less abundant and 5–8 times more powerful fast-twitch fibers that drastically respond [5,22,26,28]. These fibers grow at an alarmingly fast rate with taper [5,22,26], improving power output without a measurable change in body mass [5,22]. Improved fast-twitch fiber function may allow for a harder "push" to the finish line or improve economy (faster speed with the same amount of effort). It has recently been shown that favorable regulation of molecular hypertrophy markers, specifically in fast-twitch fibers, may support the high rate of growth in these fibers with tapering [6]. Although taper has a positive effect down to the molecular level, taper-mediated growth is only realized when volume is adequately reduced [11]. To our knowledge, data on the mechanisms of performance enhancement with tapering in strength or power athletes are not available at the muscle cell level. However, strength and power training can selectively hypertrophy fast-twitch muscle fibers [6], potentially maximizing growth adaptation before tapering ensues. Thus, tapering likely augments performance in intermittent-type athletes by a different mechanism than in endurance athletes.

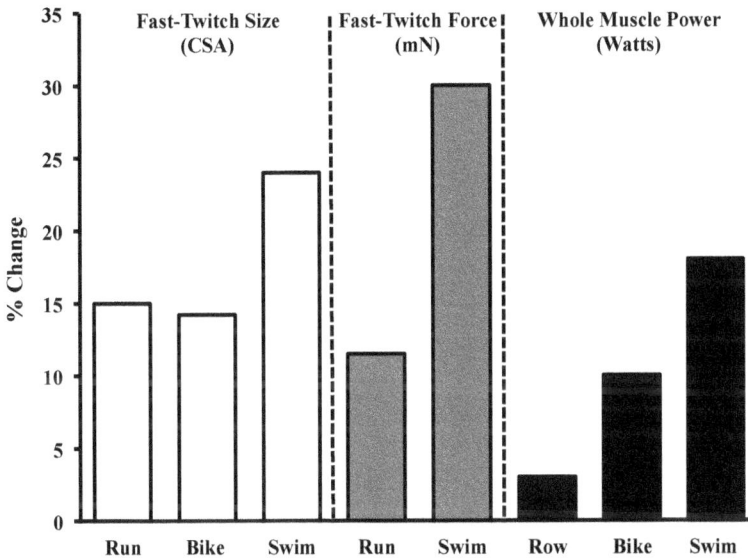

Figure 3. Skeletal muscle improvements from taper across different exercise modes and muscles. Data were derived from the following studies in order from left to right: Fast-Twitch Size-Luden *et al.* 2010 [5], Neary *et al.* 2003 [26], Trappe *et al.* 2000 [22]. Fast-Twitch Force-Luden *et al.* 2010 [5], Trappe *et al.* 2000 [22]. Whole Muscle Power-Steinacker *et al.* 2000 [21], Jeukendrup *et al.* 1992 [41], Costill *et al.* 1985 [4]. CSA = Cross Sectional Area; mN = Millinewtons.

7. How Tapering Improves Performance in Strength and Power Athletes

In the early phases of resistance training, neuromuscular mechanisms largely contribute to strength increases independent from cellular mechanisms [44,45]. It follows that strength augmentation in the early phase of taper (≤1 week) after heavy resistance training could be attributable to a reversal of neuromuscular fatigue, specifically in highly-conditioned muscle [46]. Strength improvements could also be mediated by general recovery from wear and tear caused by intense resistance training. This is evidenced by reduced circulating markers of muscle damage with taper after progressive resistance training in team sport athletes [47]. Increased muscle strength generally equates to improved power production [29,48] since power is the product of strength and speed. However, the mechanism of improved muscle function is not particularly well-documented in dedicated power athletes (e.g., competitive Olympic-style weightlifters). Regardless, total work, average peak power, repeated sprint ability, vertical jump height, and maximal power output in power-oriented athletes is observed with 10 days to three weeks of tapering [18,19,49,50]. These findings support the "rest-related augmentation" or "super-compensation" concept familiar to strength- and power-focused athletes who employ a long-term periodized training model that favors intensity over volume as competition approaches [51]. While additional mechanisms responsible for tapering's positive effect in strength, power, and team sport athletes remain to be elucidated, performance benefits are clear and tapering should be part of their training programs just as with endurance-type athletes.

8. Summary and Perspectives

The full complement of physiological effects from tapering are numerous and extend beyond the scope of this article (see Mujika *et al.* [52] and Pritchard *et al.* [17] for thorough reviews). However, the take-home points from the literature are: (1) fitness is not lost with reduced-volume training; (2) the profound effects of taper on whole muscle and fast-twitch fiber power are what appear to most greatly contribute to performance enhancement in endurance athletes; and (3) tapering is effective for improving performance in strength, power, and team sport athletes, but likely for different reasons than in endurance athletes. It should also be noted that psychological research on taper reveals that tapering improves mood state [7,21,53] and decreases perception of effort [54,55] in conjunction with improved performance. While more difficult to quantify, the psychological benefits that taper may afford prior to competition should not be understated. Nearly every well-controlled study to date on the topic of taper has shown some degree of performance enhancement so long as training volume is adequately reduced and intensity is maintained.

9. Practical Applications

The signals for adaptive processes occur during acute exercise bouts, but the actual adaptations take place during the proceeding rest periods. It follows that after a long period of chronic high-volume training that an extended period of relative rest and recovery is necessary to reap maximal performance benefits. Generally speaking, the problem with most athletes is not a lack of training rigor but demonstrating discipline and "pulling back" on training when necessary. This is evidenced by the recent findings that: (1) some elite and world-champion athletes do not adhere to the optimal tapering protocols outlined by the scientific literature and likely do not achieve true peak performance [56,57]; and (2) functional over-reaching, a common practice among recreational and elite athletes alike, may undercut the benefits of tapering [58]. Thus, tapering is adequately described by the adage "less is more" because maintained intensity with less volume yields significant performance benefits.

Author Contributions: Kevin A. Murach made substantial contributions to overall conception, drafting, and critically revising the manuscript. James R. Bagley made substantial contributions to drafting and critically revising the manuscript. Both authors approved of the final version to be published.

Conflicts of Interest: The authors declare no conflict of interest.

References

1. Spivey, J. *The Ancient Olympics*; Oxford University Press: Oxford, UK, 2004.
2. Bompa, T. *Theory and Methodology of Training: The Key to Athletic Performance*; Kendall/Hunt Publishing Company: Dubuque, IA, USA, 1983.
3. Matveev, L.P. *Periodization of Sport Training*; Fizkultura I Sport: Moskow, Russia, 1965.
4. Costill, D.; King, D.; Thomas, R.; Hagreaves, M. Effects of reduced training on muscular power in swimmers. *Phys. Sport Med.* **1985**, *13*, 94–101.
5. Luden, N.; Hayes, E.; Galpin, A.; Minchev, K.; Jemiolo, B.; Raue, U.; Trappe, T.A.; Harber, M.P.; Bowers, T.; Trappe, S. Myocellular basis for tapering in competitive distance runners. *J. Appl. Physiol.* **2010**, *108*, 1501–1509. [CrossRef] [PubMed]
6. Murach, K.; Raue, U.; Wilkerson, B.; Minchev, K.; Jemiolo, B.; Bagley, J.; Luden, N.; Trappe, S. Single muscle fiber gene expression with run taper. *PLoS ONE* **2014**, *9*. [CrossRef] [PubMed]
7. Berger, B.; Motl, R.; Butki, B.; Martin, D.; Wilkinson, J. Mood and cycling performance in response to three weeks of high-intensity, short-duration overtraining, and a two-week taper. *Sport Psychol.* **1999**, *13*, 444–457.
8. Neary, J.P.; Martin, T.P.; Reid, D.C.; Burnham, R.; Quinney, H.A. The effects of a reduced exercise duration taper programme on performance and muscle enzymes of endurance cyclists. *Eur. J. Appl. Physiol. Occup. Physiol.* **1992**, *65*, 30–36. [CrossRef] [PubMed]
9. D'Acquisto, L. Changes in aerobic power and swimming economy as a result of reduced training volume. *Biomechem. Med. Swim.* **1992**, *20*, 201–205.
10. Shepley, B.; MacDougall, J.D.; Cipriano, N.; Sutton, J.R.; Tarnopolsky, M.A.; Coates, G. Physiological effects of tapering in highly trained athletes. *J. Appl. Physiol.* **1992**, *72*, 706–711. [PubMed]
11. Harber, M.P.; Gallagher, P.M.; Creer, A.R.; Minchev, K.M.; Trappe, S.W. Single muscle fiber contractile properties during a competitive season in male runners. *Am. J. Physiol. Regul. Integr. Comp. Physiol.* **2004**, *287*, R1124–R1131. [CrossRef] [PubMed]

12. Costill, D.L.; Flynn, M.G.; Kirwan, J.P.; Houmard, J.A.; Mitchell, J.B.; Thomas, R.; Park, S.H. Effects of repeated days of intensified training on muscle glycogen and swimming performance. *Med. Sci. Sports Exerc.* **1988**, *20*, 249–254. [CrossRef] [PubMed]

13. Costill, D.L.; Thomas, R.; Roberts, R.A.; Pascoe, D.; Lambert, C.; Barr, S.; Fink, W.J. Adaptations to swimming training: Influence of training volume. *Med. Sci. Sports Exerc.* **1991**, *23*, 371–377. [CrossRef] [PubMed]

14. Mujika, I.; Padilla, S. Scientific bases for precompetition tapering strategies. *Med. Sci. Sports Exerc.* **2003**, *35*, 1182–1187. [CrossRef] [PubMed]

15. Bosquet, L.; Montpetit, J.; Arvisais, D.; Mujika, I. Effects of tapering on performance: A meta-analysis. *Med. Sci. Sports Exerc.* **2007**, *39*, 1358–1365. [CrossRef] [PubMed]

16. Wilson, J.; Wilson, G. A practical approach to the taper. *Str. Cond. J.* **2008**, *30*, 10–17. [CrossRef]

17. Pritchard, H.; Keogh, J.; Barnes, M.; McGuigan, M. Effects and mechanisms of tapering in maximizing muscular strength. *Strength Cond. J.* **2015**, *37*, 72–83. [CrossRef]

18. Zaras, N.D.; Stasinaki, A.N.; Krase, A.A.; Methenitis, S.K.; Karampatsos, G.P.; Georgiadis, G.V.; Spengos, K.M.; Terzis, G.D. Effects of tapering with light *vs.* heavy loads on track and field throwing performance. *J. Strength Cond. Res.* **2014**, *28*, 3484–3495. [CrossRef] [PubMed]

19. De Lacey, J.; Brughelli, M.; McGuigan, M.; Hansen, K.; Samozino, P.; Morin, J. The effects of tapering on power-force-velocity profiling and jump performance in professional rugby league players. *J. Strength Cond. Res.* **2014**, *28*, 3567–3570. [CrossRef] [PubMed]

20. Cavanaugh, D.; Musch, K. Arm and leg power of elite swimmers increase after taper as measired by biokinetic variable resistance machines. *J. Swim. Res.* **1989**, *5*, 7–10.

21. Steinacker, J.M.; Lormes, W.; Kellmann, M.; Liu, Y.; Reissnecker, S.; Opitz-Gress, A.; Baller, B.; Gunther, K.; Petersen, K.G.; Kallus, K.W.; *et al.* Training of junior rowers before world championships. Effects on performance, mood state and selected hormonal and metabolic responses. *J. Sports Med. Phys. Fit.* **2000**, *40*, 327–335.

22. Trappe, S.; Costill, D.; Thomas, R. Effect of swim taper on whole muscle and single muscle fiber contractile properties. *Med. Sci. Sports Exerc.* **2000**, *32*, 48–56. [CrossRef] [PubMed]

23. Houmard, J.A.; Scott, B.K.; Justice, C.L.; Chenier, T.C. The effects of taper on performance in distance runners. *Med. Sci. Sports Exerc.* **1994**, *26*, 624–631. [CrossRef] [PubMed]

24. Neary, J.P.; Bhambhani, Y.N.; McKenzie, D.C. Effects of different stepwise reduction taper protocols on cycling performance. *Can. J. Appl. Physiol.* **2003**, *28*, 576–587. [CrossRef] [PubMed]

25. Margaritis, I.; Palazzetti, S.; Rousseau, A.-S.; Richard, M.-J.; Favier, A. Antioxidant supplementation and tapering exercise improve exercise-induced antioxidant response. *J. Am. Coll. Nutr.* **2003**, *22*, 147–156. [CrossRef] [PubMed]

26. Neary, J.P.; Martin, T.P.; Quinney, H.A. Effects of taper on endurance cycling capacity and single muscle fiber properties. *Med. Sci. Sports Exerc.* **2003**, *35*, 1875–1881. [CrossRef] [PubMed]

27. Banister, E.W.; Carter, J.B.; Zarkadas, P.C. Training theory and taper: Validation in triathlon athletes. *Eur. J. Appl. Physiol. Occup. Physiol.* **1999**, *79*, 182–191. [CrossRef] [PubMed]

28. Zarkadas, P.C.; Carter, J.B.; Banister, E.W. Modelling the effect of taper on performance, maximal oxygen uptake, and the anaerobic threshold in endurance triathletes. *Adv. Exp. Med. Biol.* **1995**, *393*, 179–186. [PubMed]

29. Izquierdo, M.; Ibanez, J.; Gonzalez-Badillo, J.J.; Ratamess, N.A.; Kraemer, W.J.; Hakkinen, K.; Bonnabau, H.; Granados, C.; French, D.N.; Gorostiaga, E.M. Detraining and tapering effects on hormonal responses and strength performance. *J Strength Cond. Res.* **2007**, *21*, 768–775. [PubMed]

30. Mujika, I.; Padilla, S.; Pyne, D. Swimming performance changes during the final 3 weeks of training leading to the sydney 2000 olympic games. *Int. J. Sports. Med.* **2002**, *23*, 582–587. [CrossRef] [PubMed]

31. Vandenberghe, K.; Hespel, P.; Vanden Eynde, B.; Lysens, R.; Richter, E.A. No effect of glycogen level on glycogen metabolism during high intensity exercise. *Med. Sci. Sports Exerc.* **1995**, *27*, 1278–1283. [CrossRef] [PubMed]

32. Hargreaves, M.; Finn, J.P.; Withers, R.T.; Halbert, J.A.; Scroop, G.C.; Mackay, M.; Snow, R.J.; Carey, M.F. Effect of muscle glycogen availability on maximal exercise performance. *Eur. J. Appl. Physiol. Occup. Physiol.* **1997**, *75*, 188–192. [CrossRef] [PubMed]

33. Snyder, A.C.; Kuipers, H.; Cheng, B.; Servais, R.; Fransen, E. Overtraining following intensified training with normal muscle glycogen. *Med. Sci. Sports Exerc.* **1995**, *27*, 1063–1070. [CrossRef] [PubMed]

34. Rockwell, M.S.; Rankin, J.W.; Dixon, H. Effects of muscle glycogen on performance of repeated sprints and mechanisms of fatigue. *Int. J. Sport Nutr. Exerc. Metab.* **2003**, *13*, 1–14. [PubMed]

35. Balsom, P.D.; Gaitanos, G.C.; Soderlund, K.; Ekblom, B. High-intensity exercise and muscle glycogen availability in humans. *Acta. Physiol. Scand.* **1999**, *165*, 337–345. [CrossRef] [PubMed]

36. Bergstrom, J.; Hermansen, L.; Hultman, E.; Saltin, B. Diet, muscle glycogen and physical performance. *Acta. Physiol. Scand.* **1967**, *71*, 140–150. [CrossRef] [PubMed]

37. Sherman, W.M.; Costill, D.L.; Fink, W.J.; Miller, J.M. Effect of exercise-diet manipulation on muscle glycogen and its subsequent utilization during performance. *Int. J. Sports. Med.* **1981**, *2*, 114–118. [CrossRef] [PubMed]

38. Johns, R.A.; Houmard, J.A.; Kobe, R.W.; Hortobagyi, T.; Bruno, N.J.; Wells, J.M.; Shinebarger, M.H. Effects of taper on swim power, stroke distance, and performance. *Med. Sci. Sports. Exerc.* **1992**, *24*, 1141–1146. [CrossRef] [PubMed]

39. Van Handel, P.; Katz, A.; Troup, J.; Daniels, T.; Bradley, P. Oxygen consumption and blood lactic acid response to training and taper. *Swim. Sci.* **1988**, 269–275.

40. Halson, S.L.; Bridge, M.W.; Meeusen, R.; Busschaert, B.; Gleeson, M.; Jones, D.A.; Jeukendrup, A.E. Time course of performance changes and fatigue markers during intensified training in trained cyclists. *J. Appl. Physiol.* **2002**, *93*, 947–956. [CrossRef] [PubMed]

41. Jeukendrup, A.E.; Hesselink, M.K.; Snyder, A.C.; Kuipers, H.; Keizer, H.A. Physiological changes in male competitive cyclists after two weeks of intensified training. *Int. J. Sports Med.* **1992**, *13*, 534–541. [CrossRef] [PubMed]

42. Papoti, M.; Martins, L.E.; Cunha, S.A.; Zagatto, A.M.; Gobatto, C.A. Effects of taper on swimming force and swimmer performance after an experimental ten-week training program. *J. Strength Cond. Res.* **2007**, *21*, 538–542. [PubMed]

43. Trinity, J.D.; Pahnke, M.D.; Reese, E.C.; Coyle, E.F. Maximal mechanical power during a taper in elite swimmers. *Med. Sci. Sports Exerc.* **2006**, *38*, 1643–1649. [CrossRef] [PubMed]

44. Moritani, T.; de Vries, H.A. Neural factors *versus* hypertrophy in the time course of muscle strength gain. *Am. J. Phys. Med.* **1979**, *58*, 115–130. [PubMed]

45. Hakkinen, K.; Komi, P.V. Electromyographic changes during strength training and detraining. *Med. Sci. Sports. Exerc.* **1983**, *15*, 455–460. [CrossRef] [PubMed]

46. Hakkinen, K.; Kallinen, M.; Komi, P.V.; Kauhanen, H. Neuromuscular adaptations during short-term "normal" and reduced training periods in strength athletes. *Electromyogr. Clin. Neurophysiol.* **1991**, *31*, 35–42. [PubMed]

47. Coutts, A.; Reaburn, P.; Piva, T.J.; Murphy, A. Changes in selected biochemical, muscular strength, power, and endurance measures during deliberate overreaching and tapering in rugby league players. *Int. J. Sports Med.* **2007**, *28*, 116–124. [CrossRef] [PubMed]

48. Chtourou, H.; Anis, C.; Tarak, D.; Mohamed, D.; Behm, D.G.; Karim, C.; Nizar, S. The effect of training at the same time of day and tapering period on the dirunal variation of short exercise performances. *J. Strength Cond. Res.* **2012**, *26*, 697–708. [CrossRef] [PubMed]

49. Bishop, D.; Edge, J. The effects of a 10-day taper on repeated-sprint performance in females. *J. Sci. Med. Sport* **2005**, *8*, 200–209. [CrossRef]

50. Eliakim, A.; Nemet, D.; Bar-Sela, S.; Higer, Y.; Falk, B. Changes in circulating igf-i and their correlation with self-assessment and fitness among elite athletes. *Int. J. Sports Med.* **2002**, *23*, 600–603. [CrossRef] [PubMed]

51. Weiss, L.W.; Wood, L.E.; Fry, A.C.; Kreider, R.B.; Relyea, G.E.; Bullen, D.B.; Grindstaff, P.D. Strength/power augmentation subsequent to short-term training abstinence. *J. Strength Cond. Res.* **2004**, *18*, 765–770. [PubMed]

52. Mujika, I.; Padilla, S.; Pyne, D.; Busso, T. Physiological changes associated with the pre-event taper in athletes. *Sports Med.* **2004**, *34*, 891–927. [CrossRef] [PubMed]

53. Raglin, J.S.; Koceja, D.M.; Stager, J.M.; Harms, C.A. Mood, neuromuscular function, and performance during training in female swimmers. *Med. Sci. Sports Exerc.* **1996**, *28*, 372–377. [PubMed]

54. Flynn, M.G.; Pizza, F.X.; Boone, J.B., Jr.; Andres, F.F.; Michaud, T.A.; Rodriguez-Zayas, J.R. Indices of training stress during competitive running and swimming seasons. *Int. J. Sports Med.* **1994**, *15*, 21–26. [CrossRef] [PubMed]

55. Martin, D.T.; Scifres, J.C.; Zimmerman, S.D.; Wilkinson, J.G. Effects of interval training and a taper on cycling performance and isokinetic leg strength. *Int. J. Sports Med.* **1994**, *15*, 485–491. [CrossRef] [PubMed]

Sports **2015**, *3*, 209–218

56. Spilsbury, K.L.; Fudge, B.W.; Ingham, S.A.; Faulkner, S.H.; Nimmo, M.A. Tapering strategies in elite british endurance runners. *Eur. J. Sport. Sci.* **2014**, *15*, 1–7. [CrossRef] [PubMed]

57. Tonnesson, E.; Sylta, O.; Haugen, T.A.; Hem, E.; Svedsen, I.S.; Seiler, S. The road to gold: Training and peaking characteristics in the year prior to a gold medal endurance performance. *PLoS ONE* **2014**, *9*. [CrossRef] [PubMed]

58. Aubry, A.; Hausswirth, C.; Louis, J.; Coutts, A.J.; LE Meur, Y. Functional overreaching: The key to peak performance during the taper? *Med. Sci. Sports Exerc.* **2014**, *46*, 1769–1777. [CrossRef] [PubMed]

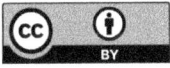

sports

MDPI

Article

Angle Specific Analysis of Side-to-Side Asymmetry in the Shoulder Rotators

Cassio V. Ruas [1,*], Ronei S. Pinto [1,†], Eduardo L. Cadore [1,†] and Lee E. Brown [2]

[1] Physical Education School, Federal University of Rio Grande do Sul, Brazil, Felizardo Street, 750—Jardim Botânico, Porto Alegre/RS 90690-200, Brazil; ronei.pinto@ufrgs.br (R.S.P.); cadoreeduardo@gmail.com (E.L.C.)

[2] Department of Kinesiology, KHS 233 800 N. State College Blvd., California State University, Fullerton 92831, CA, USA; leebrown@fullerton.edu

* Correspondence: cassiovruas@gmail.com; Tel.: +55-513-308-5894; Fax: +55-513-308-5843

† These authors contributed equally to this work.

Academic Editor: Eling de Bruin
Received: 16 July 2015; Accepted: 27 August 2015; Published: 31 August 2015

Abstract: Although side-to-side asymmetry of the shoulder rotators calculated by independent peak torque (IPT) has been used for interpretation of injury risks in athletes, it may not measure strength through the entire range of motion (ROM) tested. The aim of this study was to compare side-to-side asymmetry of the shoulder rotators between independent peak torque (IPT) and ten-degree angle specific torque (AST). Twenty healthy adult males (24.65 ± 2.4 years) performed concentric and eccentric internal rotation (IR) and external rotation (ER) of the preferred and non-preferred arms on an isokinetic dynamometer at $60°/s$ through $150°$ of total ROM. The total ROM was divided into 14 ten-degree angles of the physiological ROM from $-90°$ of ER to $60°$ of IR. Concentric and eccentric IR IPT ($10.5\% \pm 8.7\%$ and $12.1\% \pm 7.2\%$) and ER IPT ($13.6\% \pm 9.8\%$ and $8.7\% \pm 5.6\%$) were significantly less than AST at several angles ($p < 0.05$). IPT might lead to erroneous interpretations of side-to-side asymmetry in the shoulder rotators and does not represent the entire ROM tested. This information could be used to prescribe strength exercises to enhance overhead performance and reduce risk of shoulder injuries.

Keywords: angle specific torque; independent peak torque; strength imbalance; injury prevention; performance enhancement

1. Introduction

The shoulder rotator muscles are important for coordinated performance of overhead activities, such as pitching in baseball, swinging a racket in tennis or pushing against the water in swimming [1–3]. Forceful and repetitive actions in overhead sports have been associated with an increased susceptibility of shoulder rotator injuries [3,4], strength differences between external (antagonists) and internal rotator (agonists) muscles [1,3–5], and side-to-side differences between upper-limbs [2,5]. Typical shoulder strength asymmetry has been reported as an upper-limb dominance of 5%–10% measured by independent peak torque (IPT) in nonathletic and recreational-level athletes [5]. However, these IPT measurements fail to reproduce the functionality of muscles during sporting activities, because torque is not calculated through the entire range of motion (ROM), or at corresponding angles [1,6,7].

2. Context

A previous investigation has demonstrated that this can lead to misinterpretation of strength imbalance of the shoulder rotators [1]. In addition, a few studies have opted to use $5°$, $10°$, $15°$ or end of ROM angle specific torque (AST) intervals for a more accurate estimation of unilateral dynamic muscle balance of the knee or shoulder joints [1,3,4,6–9]. Dehail *et al.* [7] demonstrated there was a significant progressive decline of flexion/extension and abduction/adduction AST strength ratios as the shoulder progressed to flexion and abduction, respectively. Yildiz *et al.* [4], found that although internal rotator eccentric strength of the preferred side was greater than the non-preferred side at the end of the ROM, only the internal rotator concentric strength was greater than the non-preferred side at the beginning of the ROM. Although IPT evaluations may be more sensitive to assess muscle strength balance changes after strength rehabilitation programs [10], AST analysis has been shown to be a more appropriate tool to precisely locate potential muscle imbalances present at specific joint angles [1,6,7]. This information may be used for the prescription of strength exercises of the weak angles.

Although AST analysis has been used to measure unilateral imbalance, there is a lack of information using this approach to measure side-to-side asymmetry of the shoulder rotators. Thus, the aim of this study was to compare side-to-side asymmetry of the internal and external shoulder rotators between traditional IPT and ten-degree AST methods.

3. Method

3.1. Participants

Twenty healthy adult males (age 24.6 ± 2.4 years, body mass 81.6 ± 15.5 kg, height 175.3 ± 8.0 cm) volunteered to participate in this study. All of them participated in recreational activities (e.g., basketball, jogging, resistance training) at least once a week, and had no history of shoulder injuries in the previous six months prior to testing. Their body mass was measured using a digital scale (Model # ES200L, Ohaus, Pine Brook, NJ, USA), and height using a wall-mounted stadiometer (Seca Stadiometer, ON, Canada). All participants read and signed an informed consent form prior to participation. The study was approved by the University Institutional Review Board (HSR#130126), and the rights of the subjects were protected.

3.2. Experimental Design

Prior to testing, participants were asked about their preferred arm when throwing an object (dominance) [2]. To examine their torque capabilities, concentric isokinetic tests were performed for the internal and external shoulder rotators of the preferred and non-preferred arms. Side-to-side torque asymmetry was calculated based on these results.

3.3. Experimental Procedures

Maximal internal and external rotator concentric and eccentric strength was measured on a Biodex System 3 isokinetic dynamometer (Biodex Medical Systems, Shirley, NY, USA). Participants laid supine on the dynamometer with straps across their chest and hips to avoid additional movement. Participants grasped the lever arm of the machine and their tested arm was positioned at 90° of shoulder abduction and 90° of elbow flexion with their forearm in a neutral position in the coronal plane for alignment with the dynamometer's axis of rotation [1,11]. This position was considered 0°. Both preferred and non-preferred arms were tested.

Shoulder rotator strength was measured through 150° of total ROM, from 90° ER (−90°) to 60° IR of physiologic ROM. This ROM was chosen as it was uncomfortable for subjects to perform maximal strength beyond these limits in a pilot study. Prior to testing, participants performed a warm up of 5 submaximal repetitions at 180°/s and 3 maximal repetitions at the test speed of 60°/s for familiarization purposes. Testing consisted of 5 reciprocal concentric/concentric and 5 eccentric/eccentric maximal repetitions, with 3 min rest between modes. Preferred and non-preferred arms were assessed in random order. Participants were asked to push and pull as hard and fast as possible and verbal encouragement was provided during the test.

3.4. Outcome Measures

Maximal concentric and eccentric internal rotation (IR) and external rotation (ER) independent peak torque (IPT) were measured, as well as the angles of IPT (AIPT).

All data were collected and analyzed using custom LabVIEW Software (version 2013, National Instruments, Austin, TX, USA) and was divided into 14 ten-degree AST from $-90°$ ER to $60°$ IR of physiological ROM. Side-to-side asymmetry of the shoulder rotators for both IPT and AST were calculated as the percentage differences between the peak torque of the preferred and non-preferred arms.

3.5. Statistical Analyses

Four (IR and ER) 1×14 repeated measures ANOVAs were used to compare concentric and eccentric percentage differences between IPT and AST between arms. The effect size for each significant difference was calculated by using means (M) and standard deviations (SD) between variables to identify the magnitude and direction of the differences ($d = M_{AST} - M_{IPT}/SD_{IPT}$), in which values <0.35 were considered trivial, 0.35–0.80 small, 0.80–1.50 moderate, and >1.50 large for recreationally trained subjects [12]. All analyses were performed with SPSS version 20 (Statistical Package for Social Sciences, Chicago, IL, USA). An *a-priori* alpha level of 0.05 determined statistical significance.

4. Results

Means of concentric and eccentric IPT and AIPT of IR and ER of the preferred and non-preferred arms are presented in Table 1. Means of concentric and eccentric ten-to-ten-degree absolute AST of internal rotation (IR) and external rotation (ER) of the preferred and non-preferred arms (Table 2).

Table 1. Means ± SD of concentric and eccentric independent peak torque (IPT) and angles of independent peak torque (AIPT) of internal rotation (IR) and external rotation (ER) of the preferred and non-preferred arms.

Action	Concentric				Eccentric			
	IPT (N.m)		AIPT (°)		IPT (N.m)		AIPT (°)	
	Preferred	Non-preferred	Preferred	Non-preferred	Preferred	Non-preferred	Preferred	Non-preferred
IR	46.5 ± 16.6	44.3 ± 14.1	−35.6 ± 34.6	−33.2 ± 40.2	58.1 ± 21.0	56.9 ± 17.2	−40.9 ± 24.5	−16.3 ± 29.7
ER	42.7 ± 13.7	39.9 ± 12.1	0.7 ± 35.4	0.7 ± 31.8	52.5 ± 13.8	53.6 ± 15.1	−30.8 ± 10.8	−26.6 ± 13.9

Table 2. Means ± SD of concentric and eccentric absolute ten-to-ten-degree angle specific torque (AST) of internal rotation (IR) and external rotation (ER) of the preferred and non-preferred arms.

Angle (°)	Concentric		Eccentric	
	AST (N.m)		AST (N.m)	
	Preferred	Non-Preferred	Preferred	Non-Preferred
IR-80	38.2 ± 18.7	34.1 ± 13.0	34.4 ± 23.1	23.9 ± 24.8
IR-70	39.8 ± 17.5	37.4 ± 15.1	41.0 ± 21.2	31.3 ± 21.7
IR-60	40.9 ± 16.9	38.2 ± 15.9	47.0 ± 20.9	38.0 ± 18.8
IR-50	41.7 ± 16.8	38.0 ± 15.5	50.0 ± 20.3	45.2 ± 17.9
IR-40	41.7 ± 16.8	36.8 ± 15.0	50.9 ± 19.1	47.3 ± 18.4
IR-30	41.2 ± 15.4	37.4 ± 15.4	51.2 ± 18.5	49.6 ± 17.6
IR-20	39.6 ± 13.6	36.5 ± 14.1	50.7 ± 16.7	50.5 ± 17.3
IR-10	37.3 ± 12.1	36.6 ± 13.5	49.9 ± 15.8	50.5 ± 15.7
IR0	36.6 ± 11.6	36.8 ± 13.6	47.4 ± 16.1	50.2 ± 15.7
IR10	35.6 ± 10.7	36.3 ± 13.0	44.0 ± 15.0	49.1 ± 15.5
IR20	34.7 ± 9.9	35.8 ± 13.2	39.8 ± 14.4	47.1 ± 15.9
IR30	32.9 ± 8.9	34.9 ± 13.2	33.8 ± 14.7	42.7 ± 17.9
IR40	30.7 ± 8.5	34.0 ± 13.3	25.7 ± 14.9	35.7 ± 16.6
IR50	27.1 ± 9.1	32.3 ± 13.2	19.5 ± 11.6	24.9 ± 15.4
ER50	33.9 ± 15.1	32.8 ± 13.0	18.9 ± 14.0	19.0 ± 18.9

Table 2. *Cont.*

Angle (°)	Concentric		Eccentric	
	AST (N.m)		AST (N.m)	
	Preferred	Non-Preferred	Preferred	Non-Preferred
ER40	36.9 ± 16.2	35.2 ± 13.9	24.8 ± 17.3	27.6 ± 18.9
ER30	37.5 ± 16.0	35.7 ± 14.0	29.9 ± 17.3	33.7 ± 17.7
ER20	38.0 ± 15.2	35.9 ± 13.7	35.4 ± 15.2	37.8 ± 17.7
ER10	38.0 ± 14.0	36.0 ± 12.6	39.9 ± 14.7	40.6 ± 17.4
ER0	37.9 ± 13.0	35.9 ± 11.5	43.7 ± 14.2	44.6 ± 16.3
ER-10	38.0 ± 12.0	36.2 ± 11.5	46.5 ± 14.1	47.7 ± 16.4
ER-20	37.9 ± 11.1	36.5 ± 11.1	48.1 ± 13.2	50.8 ± 15.6
ER-30	37.8 ± 10.2	36.6 ± 10.5	50.9 ± 13.0	50.8 ± 14.1
ER-40	37.2 ± 9.6	35.6 ± 9.6	49.8 ± 12.9	48.4 ± 13.9
ER-50	35.8 ± 9.0	32.9 ± 8.4	46.4 ± 13.1	43.1 ± 13.2
ER-60	33.9 ± 9.8	29.2 ± 7.1	39.1 ± 14.3	34.4 ± 12.8
ER-70	29.1 ± 8.1	24.1 ± 6.6	29.2 ± 12.0	23.5 ± 12.7
ER-80	23.0 ± 7.9	17.2 ± 9.1	17.9 ± 10.7	14.5 ± 7.8

Concentric side-to-side IR IPT asymmetry was significantly less than AST at $-80°$ ($p = 0.018$), $-70°$ ($p = 0.045$), $-50°$ ($p = 0.029$), $-40°$ ($p = 0.018$), $-30°$ ($p = 0.016$), $-20°$ ($p = 0.027$), $40°$ ($p = 0.010$) and $50°$ ($p = 0.001$). Side-to-side ER IPT asymmetry was significantly less than AST at $50°$ ($p = 0.011$), $40°$ ($p = 0.013$) and $-80°$ ($p = 0.00017$) (Figure 1). Eccentric side-to-side IR IPT was significantly less than AST at $50°$ ($p = 0.000024$) $40°$ ($p = 0.000063$) $30°$ ($p = 0.00042$), $20°$ ($p = 0.006$), 0 ($p = 0.037$), $-70°$ ($p = 0.0013$) and $-80°$ ($p = 0.0034$). Side-to-side ER IPT was significantly less than AST at $-80°$ ($p = 0.00042$), $-70°$ ($p = 0.00026$), $-60°$ ($p = 0.0014$), $30°$ ($p = 0.0076$), $40°$ ($p = 0.0032$) and $50°$ ($p = 0.000016$) (Figure 2). Effect sizes are presented for each significant difference (Figures 1 and 2).

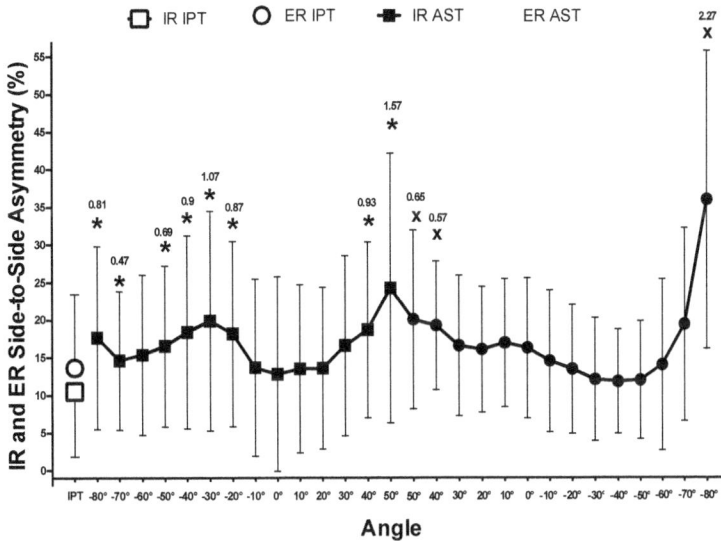

Figure 1. Means ± SD of concentric internal rotators (IR) and external rotators (ER) angle specific torque (AST) and independent peak torque (IPT) side-to-side asymmetry. * Significantly less than IR AST; x significantly less than ER AST. Effect sizes are presented for each significant difference.

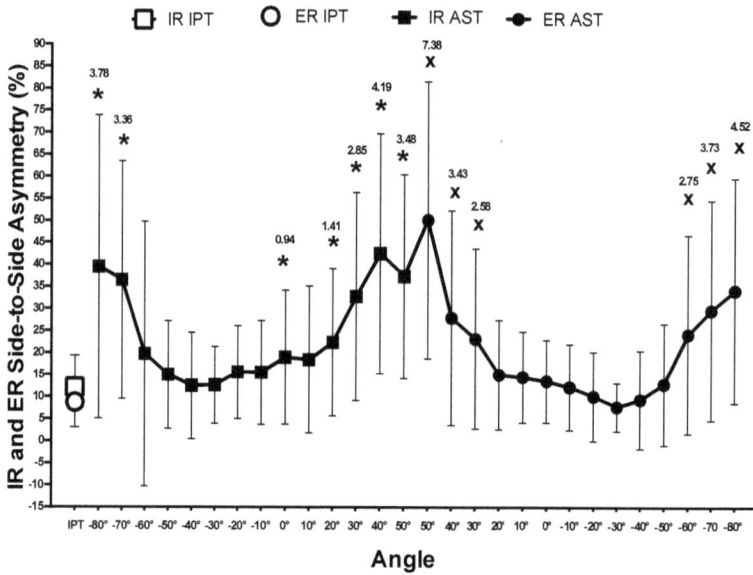

Figure 2. Means ± SD of eccentric internal rotators (IR) and external rotators (ER) angle specific torque (AST) and independent peak torque (IPT) side-to-side asymmetry. * Significantly less than IR AST; x significantly less than ER AST. Effect sizes are presented for each significant difference.

5. Discussion

The aim of this study was to compare side-to-side asymmetry of the shoulder rotators between IPT and ten-degree AST methods. Our results revealed that concentric IPT was different than AST at eight angles for IR, and three angles for ER. In addition, eccentric IPT was different than AST at seven angles for IR, and six angles for ER. ER differences were found primarily at the beginning and end points of ROM. This demonstrates that IPT might not be an accurate representation of the entire ROM tested in either testing mode. The AST values allow a more precise estimation of strength asymmetry between shoulder rotator muscles. The use of IPT alone may lead to erroneous interpretations of full ROM side-to-side strength differences.

The reliability of IPT and AST for clinical use has been questioned. Brown *et al.* [13] demonstrated a high test-retest reliability of IPT on the Biodex device over a wide velocity spectrum in the knee flexors and extensors. However, Ayala *et al.* [10] showed that this is not transferred to knee unilateral asymmetry calculations, which presented moderate reliability in strength ratios calculated by IPT, and poor reliability in ratios calculated by AST. This was also confirmed for IPT side-to-side calculations of the shoulder rotators in another recent study [14]. This might be explained by strength imbalance calculations being composed of two measurements, where each can vary in two different directions [14].

The IPT is the highest point of the torque curve across a full ROM [15]. This measurement is widely used to indicate maximum strength levels, as well as the occurrence of possible muscle strength imbalance [1,2,5,15–18]. Previous studies have widely utilized IPT as a measure to calculate side-to-side asymmetry of the shoulder internal and external rotators [2,5,14,19–22]. Ellenbecker and Davies [5] concluded that a 5%–10% IPT difference between arms is normal in recreational level upper-limb sport athletes and non-athletes. Our results are slightly outside this range, as both concentric ER and IR IPT, and eccentric IR IPT demonstrated a 10%–15% difference. This may be due to the specific method we used in our isokinetic testing. We measured participants in a supine position with their arms abducted in the frontal plane. This position was based on Forthomme *et al.* [11], which indicated that it results in greater reliability and reproducibility compared to other testing positions. To our knowledge, this position has not been used to determine side-to-side strength imbalance of the shoulder rotators in a non-athletic population. Therefore, direct comparison of our results to established normative values of previous studies [5] is problematic since shoulder asymmetry is probably position dependent as has been shown in other joints [23,24]. Nevertheless, our eccentric ER IPT results were still within the normal range suggested by Ellenbecker and Davies [5].

Our tested velocity may have also played a role in our results. Even though overhead actions such as throwing can reach speeds up to 7200°/s, especially in sports performance [4], we tested at 60°/s in order to avoid a large load range reduction during isokinetic testing, thereby significantly decreasing the total ROM available for analysis [25–27]. Brown *et al.* [26] have shown that very fast isokinetic velocities significantly affect torque patterns. This may also influence side-to-side asymmetry assessment. Greater repetitive use of the preferred arm in throwing actions in recreational and sporting activities may explain our asymmetry results [2,21]. However, previous studies have used a variety of different speeds in order to provide sport specific information about strength imbalance and injury risk in the shoulder rotators [3,4,9]. The use of a single velocity to describe angle specific strength is a limitation of our study.

The limitation of IPT is that it does not take into account the full ROM [15]. This has also been shown to affect the interpretation of shoulder rotators unilateral strength imbalance [1], and many studies have opted to use an AST approach in order to gain more specific information of joint strength imbalances [1,3,4,6–8]. We have previously demonstrated that shoulder IPT dynamic control ratios are significantly different than AST at several angles when calculated by 10° intervals over a 150° total ROM [1]. Similar to this, our present study also found significant differences between side-to-side asymmetry between concentric and eccentric IPT and AST through many ROM angles, especially for IR. In contrast, ER differences were found primarily at the beginning and end of the ROM.

The beginning shoulder ROM (cocking phase) is critical in overhead activities due to full external rotation, and superior and anterior forces being applied to the shoulder; while the end ROM (deceleration phase) requires the arm to be stopped in a short period of time from high velocities [3,4,9]. These points of the ROM have been suggested as where most imbalances may occur, leading to shoulder muscle and ligament injuries [3,4,9]. Previous reports found there were side-to-side asymmetry differences between these phases in athletes [3,4], and college students [9]. This is in agreement with our results and makes the use of AST especially important. In fact we found that eccentric ER AST at 50°, which represents the last deceleration angle at the end of the ROM, had the greatest difference and magnitude of change across all angles when compared to IPT. While ER strength is important for the preparation and deceleration phases of overhead actions, IR strength is primarily used for the acceleration phase in overhead throwing and racket sports [2,4]. A strength balance of IR and ER between upper limbs across the entire ROM, especially at the beginning and end [3–5,9], may not only help to avoid and rehabilitate injuries, but help determine performance in overhead sports [21]. Although unilateral overhead sports may result in dissimilar side-to-side differences, clinicians have assumed that peak torque value equivalency between shoulders may be used as a target for prevention and rehabilitation of injury in athletes and physically active individuals [5,21]. A strength balance between the upper limbs could be used to precisely identify where primary imbalances are present and prescribe strength exercises to diminish these differences at the affected angles. However, the greatest side-to-side asymmetry differences we found were near the extreme ranges and could be due to muscle sarcomeres being at a disadvantage on the length-tension curve and thereby generating low torques [28].

We also found that although IPT occurred at similar angles for concentric strength, they were at non-corresponding angles for eccentric strength. This could influence decision making of clinicians and physical therapists when interpreting shoulder strength results. Our results demonstrate that AST may provide a more accurate and detailed assessment of side-to-side asymmetry across the full ROM. This information can be used for the prescription of strength training programs based on bilateral equivalency for optimal performance and prevention of injury caused by repetitive sporting activities [20,21].

6. Conclusions

This study demonstrates that IPT is significantly less than AST at several angles when measuring side-to-side asymmetry of the shoulder rotators. IPT represents only one single angle across the entire ROM tested, and may occur at non-corresponding angles for eccentric strength. Therefore, AST is suggested as a new approach, which allows for measurement of the specific angles where strength differences between arms are present. This information could be used to assist in the prescription of strength training programs that focus on the precise angles where asymmetry occurs to enhance performance and reduce risk of shoulder injuries.

Author Contributions: Cassio V. Ruas, Ronei S. Pinto and Lee E. Brown were involved in study design and data interpretation. Cassio V. Ruas and Lee E. Brown were involved in data collection. Cassio V. Ruas, Ronei S. Pinto, Eduardo L. Cadore and Lee E. Brown were involved in manuscript writing and revision.

Conflicts of Interest: The authors declare no conflict of interest.

References

1. Ruas, C.V.; Pinto, R.S.; Hafenstine, R.W.; Pereira, M.C.; Brown, L.E. Specific joint angle assessment of the shoulder rotators. *Isokinet. Exerc. Sci.* **2014**, *22*, 197–204.
2. Gulick, D.T.; Dustman, C.S.; Ossowski, L.L.; Outslay, M.D.; Thomas, C.P.; Trucano, S. Side dominance does not affect dynamic control strength ratios in the shoulder. *Isokinet. Exerc. Sci.* **2001**, *9*, 79–84.
3. Ng, G.Y.; Lam, P.C. A study of antagonist/agonist isokinetic work ratios of shoulder rotators in men who play badminton. *J. Orthop. Sports Phys. Ther.* **2002**, *32*, 399–404. [CrossRef] [PubMed]
4. Yildiz, Y.; Aydin, T.; Sekir, U.; Kiralp, M.Z.; Hazneci, B.; Kalyon, T.A. Shoulder terminal range eccentric antagonist/concentric agonist strength ratios in overhead athletes. *Scand. J. Med. Sci. Sports* **2006**, *16*, 174–180. [CrossRef] [PubMed]
5. Ellenbecker, T.S.; Davies, G.J. The application of isokinetics in testing and rehabilitation of the shoulder complex. *J. Athl. Train.* **2000**, *35*, 338–350. [PubMed]
6. Kellis, E.; Katis, A. Quantification of functional knee flexor to extensor moment ratio using isokinetics and electromyography. *J. Athl. Train.* **2007**, *42*, 477–485. [PubMed]
7. Dehail, P.; Gagnon, D.; Noreau, L.; Nadeau, S. Assessment of agonist-antagonist shoulder torque ratios in individuals with paraplegia: A new interpretative approach. *Spinal Cord.* **2008**, *46*, 552–558. [CrossRef] [PubMed]
8. Evangelidis, P.E.; Pain, M.T.; Folland, J. Angle-specific hamstring-to-quadriceps ratio: A comparison of football players and recreationally active males. *J. Sports Sci.* **2015**, *33*, 309–319. [CrossRef] [PubMed]
9. Scoville, C.R.; Arciero, R.A.; Taylor, D.C.; Stoneman, P.D. End range eccentric antagonist/concentric agonist strength ratios: A new perspective in shoulder strength assessment. *J. Orthop. Sports Phys. Ther.* **1997**, *25*, 203–207. [CrossRef] [PubMed]
10. Ayala, F.; De Ste Croix, M.; Sainz de Baranda, P.; Santonja, F. Absolute reliability of hamstring to quadriceps strength imbalance ratios calculated using peak torque, joint angle-specific torque and joint rom-specific torque values. *Int. J. Sports Med.* **2012**, *33*, 909–916. [CrossRef] [PubMed]
11. Forthomme, B.; Dvir, Z.; Crielaard, J.M.; Croisier, J.L. Isokinetic assessment of the shoulder rotators: A study of optimal test position. *Clin. Physiol. Funct. Imaging* **2011**, *31*, 227–232. [CrossRef] [PubMed]
12. Rhea, M.R. Determining the magnitude of treatment effects in strength training research through the use of the effect size. *J. Strength Cond. Res.* **2004**, *18*, 918–920. [PubMed]
13. Brown, L.E.; Whitehurst, M.; Bryant, J.R.; Buchalter, D.N. Reliability of the biodex system 2 isokinetic dynamometer concentric mode. *Isokinet. Exerc. Sci.* **1993**, *3*, 160–163.
14. Edouard, P.; Codine, P.; Samozino, P.; Bernard, P.L.; Herisson, C.; Gremeaux, V. Reliability of shoulder rotators isokinetic strength imbalance measured using the biodex dynamometer. *J. Sci. Med. Sport* **2013**, *16*, 162–165. [CrossRef] [PubMed]

15. Brown, L.E.; Weir, J.P. Asep procedures recommendation i: Accurate assessment of muscular strength and power. *J. Exerc. Physiol. Online* **2001**, *4*, 1–21.
16. Ruas, C.V.; Minozzo, F.; Pinto, M.D.; Brown, L.E.; Pinto, R.S. Lower-extremity strength ratios of professional soccer players according to field position. *J. Strength Cond. Res.* **2015**, *29*, 1220–1226. [CrossRef] [PubMed]
17. Ruas, C.V.; Pinto, M.D.; Brown, L.; Minozzo, F.; Mil-Homens, P.; Pinto, R.S. The association between conventional and dynamic control knee strength ratios in elite soccer players. *Isokinet. Exerc. Sci.* **2015**, *23*, 1–12.
18. Brown, L.E.; Sjostrom, T.; Comeau, M.J.; Whitehurst, M.; Greenwood, M.; Findley, B.W. Kinematics of biophysically asymmetric limbs within rate of velocity development. *J. Strength Cond. Res.* **2005**, *19*, 298–301. [PubMed]
19. Hurd, W.J.; Kaplan, K.M.; ElAttrache, N.S.; Jobe, F.W.; Morrey, B.F.; Kaufman, K.R. A profile of glenohumeral internal and external rotation motion in the uninjured high school baseball pitcher, part ii: Strength. *J. Athl. Train.* **2011**, *46*, 289–295. [PubMed]
20. Codine, P.; Bernard, P.L.; Pocholle, M.; Benaim, C.; Brun, V. Influence of sports discipline on shoulder rotator cuff balance. *Med. Sci. Sports Exerc.* **1997**, *29*, 1400–1405. [CrossRef] [PubMed]
21. Perrin, D.H.; Robertson, R.J.; Ray, R.L. Bilateral lsokinetic peak torque, torque acceleration energy, power, and work relationships in athletes and nonathletes. *J. Orthop. Sports Phys. Ther.* **1987**, *9*, 184–189. [CrossRef] [PubMed]
22. Sirota, S.C.; Malanga, G.A.; Eischen, J.J.; Laskowski, E.R. An eccentric- and concentric-strength profile of shoulder external and internal rotator muscles in professional baseball pitchers. *Am. J. Sports Med.* **1997**, *25*, 59–64. [CrossRef] [PubMed]
23. Findley, B.W.; Brown, L.E.; Whitehurst, M.; Keating, T.; Murray, D.P.; Gardner, L.M. The influence of body position on load range during isokinetic knee extension/flexion. *J. Sport Sci. Med.* **2006**, *5*, 400–406.
24. Findley, B.W.; Brown, L.E.; Whitehurst, M.; Gilbert, R.; Groo, D.R.; O'neal, J. Sitting *vs.* Standing isokinetic trunk extension and flexion performance differences. *J. Strength Cond Res.* **2000**, *14*, 310–315.
25. Brown, L.E.; Whitehurst, M.; Gilbert, R.; Buchalter, D.N. The effect of velocity and gender on load range during knee extension and flexion exercise on an isokinetic device. *J. Orthop. Sports Phys. Ther.* **1995**, *21*, 107–112. [CrossRef] [PubMed]
26. Brown, L.E.; Whitehurst, M.; Findley, B.W.; Gilbert, R.; Buchalter, D.N. Isokinetic load range during shoulder rotation exercise in elite male junior tennis players. *J. Strength Cond. Res.* **1995**, *9*, 160–164.
27. Brown, L.E.; Whitehurst, M.; Findley, B.W.; Gilbert, R.; Groo, D.R.; Jimenez, J.A. Effect of repetitions and gender on acceleration range of motion during knee extension on an isokinetic device. *J. Strength Cond. Res.* **1998**, *12*, 222–225.
28. Huxley, A.F.; Niedergerke, R. Structural changes in muscle during contraction. *Nature* **1954**, *173*, 971–973. [CrossRef] [PubMed]

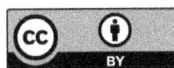

![sports logo] *sports*

MDPI

Article

Relationship of Two Vertical Jumping Tests to Sprint and Change of Direction Speed among Male and Female Collegiate Soccer Players

Isaiah T. McFarland [1,†], J. Jay Dawes [1,*,†], Craig L. Elder [1,†] and Robert G. Lockie [2,†]

1   Department of Health Sciences, University of Colorado-Colorado Springs, 1420 Austin Bluffs Blvd,
    Colorado Springs, CO 80923, USA; imcfarland@uccs.edu (I.T.M.); celder@uccs.edu (C.L.E.)
2   Department of Kinesiology, California State University, Northridge, 18111 Nordhoff St, Northridge,
    CA 91330-8272, USA; robert.lockie@csun.edu
*   Correspondence: jdawes@uccs.edu; Tel.: +1-719-255-3000 (ext. 7529)
†   These authors contributed equally to this work.

Academic Editor: Lee E. Brown
Received: 12 December 2015; Accepted: 3 February 2016; Published: 16 February 2016

Abstract: In collegiate level soccer acceleration, maximal velocity and agility are essential for successful performance. Power production is believed to provide a foundation for these speed qualities. The purpose of this study was to determine the relationship of change of direction speed, acceleration, and maximal velocity to both the counter movement jump (CMJ) and squat jump (SJ) in collegiate soccer players. Thirty-six NCAA Division II soccer players (20 males and 16 females) were tested for speed over 10 and 30 m, CODS (T-test, pro agility) and power (CMJ, SJ). Independent t-tests ($p \leqslant 0.05$) were used to derive gender differences, and Pearson's correlations ($p \leqslant 0.05$) calculated relationships between the different power and speed tests. Female subjects displayed moderate-to-strong correlations between 30 m, pro agility and T-test with the CMJ ($r = -0.502$ to -0.751), and SJ ($r = -0.502$ to -0.681). Moderate correlations between 10 and 30 m with CMJ ($r = -0.476$ and -0.570) and SJ ($r = -0.443$ and -0.553, respectively) were observed for males. Moderate to strong relationships exist between speed and power attributes in both male and female collegiate soccer players, especially between CMJ and maximal velocity. Improving stretch shortening cycle (SSC) utilization may contribute to enhanced sport-specific speed.

Keywords: soccer; agility; power; change of direction speed; linear speed

1. Introduction

The ability to start, stop and change directions rapidly and efficiently is essential for success in most team sports [1–4]. This is especially true for sports that require intermittent repeat sprints, such as soccer. Within a 90 min soccer match, players may perform over 600 changes of direction [5] and numerous linear sprints ranging in distance between 1.5 and 105 m. These high-intensity speed bouts are critical to the game's outcome and ultimately a team's success [2,6,7].

There appears to be a significant relationship between speed and one's ability exert force rapidly [8]. Subsequently, the countermovement vertical jump (CMJ) and squat jump (SJ) are two commonly used field tests to assess lower-body power [9]. Numerous studies indicate that a significant relationship exists between sprint acceleration performance and SJ height. Similarly, the CMJ has been shown to demonstrate moderately strong correlations to maximal sprint velocity [10,11].

Several studies have also revealed an association between measures of leg power and change of direction speed (CODS) [12–15]; however, these results have been inconsistent. In a study conducted by Fatih (2009) [12], moderate relationships between vertical jump performance and CODS (Hexagonal Obstacle Test) were discovered among both adolescent boys ($p < 0.05$) and girls ($p < 0.01$). Barnes *et al.*

(2007) [13] found the CMJ was a significant predictor of agility performance (34% variance) among female collegiate volleyball players in which the athletes performed four 5 m sprints with three 180° turns. Lockie *et al.* (2014) [16] investigated the relationship between unilateral jump performance and multi-directional speed in male team-sport athletes ($n = 30$). Left leg vertical jump (LVJ) had no notable correlations with T-test scores, however right leg vertical jump (RVJ) did ($r = -0.380$ to -0.512, $p \leqslant 0.05$). Left-leg standing broad-jump (SBJ) and lateral jump (LJ) correlated with both the T-test and 505 agility tests ($r = -0.370$ to -0.729, $p \leqslant 0.05$). This demonstrates a relationship between CODS and power in male athletes as well, however the existence of such relationships seem to be dependent on the CODS test being performed, as well as whether a jump test is conducted bilaterally or unilaterally. These varied results may be due to the diversity in both study populations and different CODS tests performed.

It is also important to determine whether there are gender differences in lower-body power measured by jump performance, and linear speed and CODS. Possible physiological and biomechanical differences that may influence the strength of the relationship between power production and speed qualities include muscular strength, technique, motor abilities, and anatomical difference (*i.e.*, Q-angle, femoral notch width) [17,18]. The relationships between leg power, as measured by the SJ and CMJ, and linear speed and CODS requires further investigation in collegiate soccer players, both from a performance and gender perspective.

Therefore, the purpose for this study is to investigate the production of power as measured by the SJ and CMJ and their relationship to the performance of acceleration, maximal velocity, and CODS among NCAA Division 2 male and female soccer players [9]. Please note that as SJ and CMJ are not direct measures of power, jump height is a measurable result of power production that is highly applicable to performance in many sports, and serves as an easy, cost effective field assessment for strength and sport coaches. Sport and strength coaches could design efficient and relevant skill testing/training regimens to better improve performance qualities by incorporating power tests that are more strongly associated with acceleration, maximal velocity and CODS as independent speed attributes.

2. Materials and Methods

2.1. Subjects

Performance testing data for thirty-six (Male = 20, Female = 16) NCAA Division II soccer players was used for this analysis. All subjects were between 18 and 23 years of age, a mean height of 67.71 ± 3.50 cm for males and 64.21 ± 2.68 cm for females, and mean weight of 75.80 ± 7.73 kg for males and 62.37 ± 7.07 kg for females. Institutional Review Board approval was obtained to conduct data analysis on this archival data set. Nonetheless, the study still conformed to the recommendations of the Declaration of Helsinki. All testing was performed indoors on a hardwood basketball court in single session.

2.2. Procedures

Two different pre-season testing sessions were performed in close proximity, one for males and one for females. Athletes were requested to wear clothing that would not restrict movement (*i.e.*, shorts, sweats, and athletic wear) and to wear a good pair of athletic shoes. All testing was conducted indoors on a hardwood basketball court in order to maintain a consistent testing surface and eliminate extraneous variables, such as wind or rain that may confound testing results. After anthropometric information was measured and recorded for each athlete, a standardized warm-up, led by a certified strength and conditioning specialist, was conducted prior to testing. This warm-up lasted approximately 10 min and consisted of light walking, jogging, and dynamic stretching. Once the warm-up was completed the testing began. All tests were performed on the same day under the direction of the university's athletic performance staff. Testing order was arranged in a manner to ensure that one test would interfere with the performance of another test. Subjects also received an oral and visual demonstration of the proper techniques required to successfully complete each test before they were asked to perform them. Subjects were then allowed up to three sub-maximal trials to practice technique. Once the submaximal trials were completed the athletes performed each assessment. The SJ and CMJ were performed at the same time in a randomized fashion. Immediately following these measures the athletes were randomly assigned to either perform the pro-agility or T-test. The order of both agility tests were randomized in order to reduce any order effects, as well as maximize the allotted amount of time to conduct the testing session. Once all CODS tests were completed the athletes performed the 30 m sprint.

2.3. Anthropometric Data

Anthropometric information, including height (cm) and weight (kg) measurements were collected using standard procedures on a doctors beam scale (Cardinal; Detecto Scale Co, Webb City, MO, USA).

2.4. Squat Jump and Countermovement Jump Test

Vertical jump height for the SJ and CMJ was measured using an electronic jump mat (Just Jump, ProBotics Inc., Huntsville, AL, USA). This device calculates vertical jump height by measuring flight time against gravity (9.81 m/s), and when compared to the jump and reach Vertec measuring device the Just Jump Mat system has been shown to be a valid method ($R = 0.906$) for measuring vertical jump height [19]. All athletes were instructed to step on the mat, place their hands on their hips, and when ready, jump as high as possible. For the SJ the athletes were further instructed to lower themselves to the bottom of a jumping position so that an angle of approximately 90° knee flexion was achieved, hold for a minimum of 2 s, and proceeding through a strictly concentric jumping motion. Each athlete performed the SJ and CMJ in a randomized order, recording the best of 3 attempts for each. The Sayers power equation (Peak power (Watts) = 60.7 × jump height (cm) + 45.3 × body mass (kg)—2055) was used to estimate total power output in watts. This information was normalized for each athlete by dividing power output by total body mass to determine the power to weight ratio (P:W) for SJ and CMJ.

2.5. Pro-Agility Shuttle

Athletes stood on the starting line and on the "go" command sprinted 5 yards to the right, touch the designated line with the right foot, immediately sprinted 10 yards to the left and touched the designated line with the left foot, then completed the shuttle by sprinting through the start line. Similar to previous research, a hand held stopwatch was used to record the time required to complete this test, with times rounded to the nearest 0.10 s, and the best of three trials was recorded [20].

2.6. T-Test

The T-test used the protocol outlined by Paulo *et al.* [21]. Time required to complete each trial was measured with a Speed Trap II (TC-System, Brower Timing Systems, Draper, UT, USA) automatic timing device. This device was set up on the starting line. To perform the test athletes assumed a staggered stance just behind the starting line. The timer started when the crossed the infrared beam and stopped when they crossed the beam a second time upon returning to the start line. The best of three trials was recorded, and rounded to the nearest 0.10 of a second.

2.7. Thirty Meter Sprint Test

Sprint speed (10 m and 30 m) were measured using an electronic timing system (TC-System, Brower Timing Systems, Draper, UT, USA). The 10 m time provided a measure of acceleration, while 30 m time measured maximal velocity sprinting. Each athlete was allowed three attempts with the best time being recorded to the nearest 0.10 s. using a staggered stance, athletes positioned themselves behind the starting line with their front foot on a weight sensitive timing pad. The timer started when the athlete stepped the pad, and stopped after sprinting the full 30 m distance. Timing gates were set at both the 10 and 30 m marks in order to measure both acceleration and maximal velocity. The best of three trials was recorded, and rounded to the nearest 0.10 of a second.

2.8. Statistical Analysis

Collected data was entered into a computer file suitable for statistical analysis using the Statistics Package for Social Sciences (Version 23.0; IBM Corporation, New York, NY, USA). A descriptive statistical analysis was conducted to determine the mean scores and standard deviations for the total sample on all anthropometric and performance scores. Between groups comparisons were analyzed using a series of independent *t*-tests. Pearson's correlations were also performed to determine the relationships between all four speed and CODS measures, and the squat jump and countermovement jump tests. Relationships between all speed and CODs and estimated peak power in watts, in relative an absolute terms were investigated ($p = 0.05$). In addition, significance level was set at $p \leqslant 0.05$ for all calculations and r-values were interpreted as weak ($\leqslant 0.39$), moderate ($\leqslant 0.40$–0.69) or strong ($\geqslant 0.70$) [22].

3. Results

Descriptive statistics for both groups are displayed in Table 1. When separated by gender, female collegiate soccer players displayed strong correlations between (PAPw) and CODS, as well as the 30 m sprint (Table 2). Male players displayed moderate correlations between PAPw and both the 10 and 30 m sprints, but not CODS. For the females, the 30 m was almost as strongly related to CMJ as SJ, and CMJ displayed considerably stronger relationships to the pro-agility shuttle and T-test than did SJ. In male soccer players, a slightly stronger correlation was seen between CMJ and both the 10 and 30 m compared to the SJ. The power to weight (P:W) ratios calculated for both the CMJ and SJ displayed moderate to strong correlations with the various speed qualities, however they were inconsistent across the different tests and gender.

Table 1. Descriptive statistics.

Performance Test	Gender (M = 20; F = 16)	Mean ± SD
SJ (cm)	F	40.15 ± 4.66
	M	54.81 ± 6.70
CMJ (cm)	F	41.85 ± 4.98
	M	58.47 ± 6.53
10 m	F	1.92 ± 0.31
	M	1.63 ± 0.12
30 m	F	4.78 ± 0.22
	M	4.16 ± 0.14
Pro Agility (s)	F	5.36 ± 0.18
	M	4.64 ± 0.25
T-test (s)	F	11.920 ± 0.56
	M	10.22 ± 0.41
PAPw (CMJ)	F	3310.54 ± 474.11
	M	4927.71 ± 567.16
P:W (CMJ)	F	53.08 ± 5.03
	M	86.13 ± 5.17
PAPw (SJ)	F	3207.43 ± 448.91
	M	4705.703 ± 616.91
P:W (SJ)	F	51.44 ± 4.60
	M	62.10 ± 4.96

Notes: SJ = squat jump; CMJ = counter movement jump; PAPw = peak anaerobic power in watts; P:W = power to watt ratio.

Table 2. Correlations (r-values) of selected measures of power with acceleration, maximal speed and CODS by gender.

Performance Test	10 m (Acceleration)		30 m (Max Speed)		Pro Agility		T-Test	
	M	**F**	**M**	**F**	**M**	**F**	**M**	**F**
SJ	−0.44	−0.31	−0.55 *	−0.68 *	−0.32	−0.50 *	−0.23	−0.68 *
CMJ	−0.47 *	−0.22	−0.57 *	−0.67 *	−0.30	−0.58	−0.16	−0.76 *
PAPw (CMJ)	−0.49 *	−0.53 *	−0.48 *	−0.53 *	0.03	−0.50 *	0.02	−0.46
P:W (CMJ)	−0.30	−0.10	−0.45 *	−0.63 *	−0.45 *	−0.60 *	−0.25	−0.79 *
PAPw (SJ)	−0.43	−0.61 *	−0.44	−0.53 *	0.01	−0.44	−0.02	−0.41
P:W (SJ)	−0.32	−0.23	−0.48 *	−0.65 *	−0.48 *	−0.53 *	−0.34	−0.72 *

Notes: SJ = squat jump; CMJ = counter movement jump; PAPw = peak anaerobic power in watts; P:W = power to watt ratio; *: $p \leqslant 0.05$.

4. Discussion

In the sport of soccer, power has been linked to the ability to accelerate, achieve maximal velocity and effectiveness in COD tasks [1–4,10–15]. By definition, acceleration refers to the capacity to rapidly increase speed [10]. As such, starting strength, or the ability to rapidly generate working force, is a major factor [23]. This elicits the functional significance of lower-body power in the production of acceleration. Compared to the CMJ, slightly stronger correlations have been found between SJ and acceleration over distances of 0–20 m ($r = −0.43$ to $−0.76$, respectively) [12–14]. This was further reinforced by our findings with female soccer players, though the correlation between CMJ was only marginally lower ($r = −0.317$ SJ, $r = −0.222$ CMJ, $p \leqslant 0.05$). However, for the males SJ had a slightly lower correlation with acceleration compared to CMJ ($r = −0.443$ SJ, $−0.476$ CMJ $p \leqslant 0.05$). Results showing stronger correlations between SJ and acceleration may be due to the fact that adequate starting strength is necessary to initiate acceleration and overcome inertia and does not rely as heavily on the SSC due to a static starting position [24]. However, in the sport of soccer, players are often already in motion when a sprint is initiated [2]. In this case, the SSC is already contributing to force generation during a moving or rolling start. This means that mechanically it is more similar to a maximal sprint where short ground contact time and the assistance of stored elastic energy as seen in the CMJ is now a contributing factor. Given this knowledge, it may be more beneficial for coaches to focus on assessment tests and exercise selections, which improve the SSC utilization when working with collegiate soccer players. It should be considered that other variances in acceleration performance outcomes including maximal leg strength and technique are unaccounted for and may have a strong influence on such performance outcomes [25].

Strong correlations were shown between maximal velocity and power output in both male and female soccer players in this study. For males, the CMJ had a slightly stronger correlation when compared to SJ. For the females the opposite was seen, with SJ showing slightly stronger correlations with maximal velocity than CMJ. This is in agreement with previous research studies [12,13]. This further indicates the possible benefits of maximal velocity obtained from improved utilization of the SSC.

When considering gender differences the test results and the training and assessment indications vary for males and females. Female soccer players demonstrated that the CMJ was more strongly correlated with CODS ($r = −0.58$ Pro Agility, $r = −0.76$ T-test, $p \leqslant 0.05$). In the males, we observed only minor relationships between CMJ and CODS ($p > 0.05$). This is similar to the results seen by Barnes *et al.* (2007). Barnes *et al.* (2007) discovered strong correlations between CMJ and CODS utilizing short sprints and 180° turns in female athletes. Furthermore, there appears to be relatively consistent findings showing CMJ as a good predictor of CODS performance in females [10]. It is difficult to determine if the observed differences are due to gender or the specific tests used in the research studies. For example, a contributing factor could be the volume of linear sprinting that exists within a COD test. COD assessments that feature more linear sprinting may reduce the influence of COD ability, and rely more heavily on characteristics important for linear speed, such as the SSC qualities of muscles [26,27]. Future research into the relationship between leg power, and a measure such as exit velocity from a COD, would be beneficial [27–30].

It may be of note that the authors of this paper decided to focus on the SJ and CMJ heights achieved due to their practical applications. The results of this study may only be applicable to division II collegiate soccer players specifically. Other weaknesses of this study include the sample size being limited to division II varsity soccer teams for only one university, as well as the exclusion of other power tests such as weighted jumps squats or drop jumps. Other such tests could be indicative of other power categories such as reactive strength, and their impact on the development of the various speed qualities pertinent to successful performance in soccer.

5. Conclusions

The results of this study indicate moderate to strong relationships between speed and power attributes in both male and female collegiate soccer players, especially between CMJ and maximal velocity. By including exercises that improve SSC utilization when training soccer players, improved development of acceleration, CODS, and especially that of maximal velocity may occur. If time restraints during testing sessions are also an issue, as they often are, the coach may choose to only use CMJ for power testing as it seems to have stronger correlations with respect to all of the above speed attributes pertinent for soccer performance. It is unclear as to whether or not the results of this study would apply to all soccer populations as our study sample consisted of male and female division II collegiate soccer players. Future studies observing different populations and competitive levels within the soccer community will further enhance our knowledge regarding the relationships between power production and various speed performance. It may also be advantageous to investigate power production differences and their relationships between different field positions (*i.e.*, defenders, midfielders, forwards and goalkeepers). Also, further investigation into the correlations witnessed between both P:W and PAPw may contribute to the understanding of physiological and performance relationships between power production and speed qualities in field sport athletes. Collectively, this knowledge will further benefit sport specific training and player development.

Author Contributions: Isaiah T. McFarland, Craig L. Elder and Robert G. Lockie were involved in data interpretation, and manuscript writing. J. Jay Dawes was involved in study design, data collection, data interpretation, and manuscript writing.

Conflicts of Interest: The authors declare no conflict of interest.

References

1. Kutlu, M.; Yapici, H.; Yoncalik, O.; Celik, S. Comparison of a new test for agility and skill in soccer with other agility tests. *J. Hum. Kinet.* **2012**, *33*, 143–150. [CrossRef] [PubMed]
2. Little, T.; Williams, A. Specificity of acceleration, maximum speed and agility in professional soccer players. *J. Strength Cond. Res.* **2005**, *19*, 76–78. [PubMed]
3. Lockie, R.; Shultz, A.; Callaghan, S.; Jeffriess, M.; Berry, S. Reliability and validity of a new change-of-direction speed for field based sports; the change-of-direction and acceleration tests (CODAT). *J. Sports Sci. Med.* **2013**, *12*, 88–96. [PubMed]
4. Sporis, G.; Jukic, I.; Milanovic, L.; Vucetic, V. Reliability and factorial validity of agility tests for soccer players. *J. Strength Cond. Res.* **2010**, *24*, 679–686. [CrossRef] [PubMed]
5. Bloomfield, J.; Polman, R.; O'Donoghue, P. Physical demands of different positions in FA premier league soccer. *J. Sports Sci. Med.* **2007**, *21*, 63–70.
6. Faude, O.; Koch, T.; Meyer, T. Straight sprinting is the most frequent action in goal situations in professional football. *J. Sports Sci.* **2012**, *30*, 625–631. [CrossRef] [PubMed]
7. Rienzi, E.; Drust, B.; Reilly, T.; Carter, J.E.; Martin, A. Investigation of anthropometric and work-rate profiles of elite South American international soccer players. *J. Sports Med. Phys. Fit.* **2000**, *40*, 162–169.
8. Bompa, T.; Buzzichelli, C. Periodization as Planning and Programming of Sport Training. In *Periodization Training for Sports*, 3rd ed.; Human Kinetics: Champaigne, IL, USA, 2015.

9. Cardinale, M.; Newton, R.; Kazunori, N. Speed and Agility Assessment. In *Strength and Conditioning: Biological Principles and Practical Applications*; Wiley-Blackwell: West Sussex, UK, 2011; pp. 259–277.

10. Shalfawi, S.; Enoksen, E.; Tonnessen, E. The relationship between measures of sprinting, aerobic fitness, and lower body strength and power in well trained female soccer players. *Int. J. Appl. Sports Sci.* **2014**, *26*, 18–25.

11. Cronin, J.; Hansen, K. Strength and power predictors of sports speed. *J. Strength Cond. Res.* **2005**, *19*, 349–357. [PubMed]

12. Fatih, H. The relationship of jumping and agility performance in children. *Sci. Mov. Health* **2009**, *9*, 415–419.

13. Barnes, J.; Schilling, B.; Falvo, M.; Weiss, L.; Creasy, A.; Fry, A. Relationship of jumping and agility performance in female volleyball athletes. *J. Strength Cond. Res.* **2007**, *21*, 1192–1196. [PubMed]

14. McCormick, B. The relationship between lateral movement and power in female adolescent basketball play. *Arena J. Phys. Act.* **2014**, *3*, 13–28.

15. Lockie, R.; Shultz, A.; Callaghan, S.; Jeffries, M.; Luczo, T. Contribution of leg power to multidirectional speed in Field sport athletes. *J. Aust. Strength Cond.* **2014**, *22*, 16–24.

16. Lockie, R.G.; Callaghan, S.J.; Berry, S.P.; Cooke, E.R.; Jordan, C.A.; Luczo, T.M.; Jeffriess, M.D. Relationship between unilateral jumping ability and asymmetry on multidirectional speed in team-sport athletes. *J. Strength Cond. Res.* **2014**, *28*, 3557–3566. [CrossRef] [PubMed]

17. Hewett, T.E.; Ford, K.R.; Myer, G.D.; Wanstrath, K.; Scheper, M. Gender differences in hip adduction motion and torque during a single-leg agility maneuver. *J. Orthop. Res.* **2006**, *24*, 416–421. [CrossRef] [PubMed]

18. Grandstrand, S.L.; Pfeiffer, R.P.; Sabick, M.B.; de Beliso, M.; Shea, K.G. The effects of a commercially available warm-up program on landing mechanics in female youth soccer players. *J. Strength Cond. Res.* **2006**, *20*, 331–335. [PubMed]

19. Leard, J.S.; Cirillo, M.A.; Katsnelson, E.; Kimiatek, D.A.; Miller, T.W.; Trebincevic, K.; Garbalosa, J.C. Validity of two alternative systems for measuring vertical jump height. *J. Strength Cond. Res.* **2007**, *21*, 1296–1299. [PubMed]

20. Dupler, T.; Amonette, W.; Coleman, A.; Hoffman, J.; Wenzel, T. Arthroscopic and performance differences among high-school football players. *J. Strength Cond. Res.* **2010**, *24*, 1975–1982. [CrossRef] [PubMed]

21. Pauole, K.; Madole, K.; Garhammer, J.; Lacourse, M.; Rozenek, R. Reliability and validity of the T-test as a measure of agility, leg power, and leg speed in college-aged men and women. *J. Strength Cond. Res.* **2000**, *14*, 443–450.

22. Cohen, J.; Cohen, P.; West, S.G.; Aiken, L.S. *Applied Multiple Regression/Correlation Analysis for the Behavioral Sciences*; Routledge: London, UK, 2013.

23. Verkoshansky, Y.; Siff, M. Programming and Organization of Training. In *Supertraining*, 6th ed.; Ultimate Athlete Concepts: Muskegon Heights, MI, USA, 2009; p. 109.

24. Henricks, B. A comparison of strength qualities and their influence on sprint acceleration. *J. Aust. Strength Cond.* **2014**, *22*, 77–84.

25. Lockie, R.G.; Murphy, A.J.; Knight, T.J.; de Jonge, X.A.J. Factors that differentiate acceleration ability in field sport athletes. *J. Strength Cond. Res.* **2011**, *25*, 2704–2714. [CrossRef] [PubMed]

26. Nimphius, S.; McGuigan, M.; Newton, R. Relationship between strength, power, speed, and change of direction performance in female softball players. *J. Strength Cond. Res.* **2010**, *24*, 885–895. [CrossRef]

27. Sayers, M.G. Influence of test distance on change of direction speed test results. *J. Strength Cond. Res.* **2015**, *29*, 2412–2416. [CrossRef] [PubMed]

28. Spiteri, T.; Cochrane, J.L.; Hart, N.H.; Haff, G.G.; Nimphius, S. Effect of strength on plant foot kinetics and kinematics during a change of direction task. *Eur. J. Sport Sci.* **2013**, *13*, 646–652. [CrossRef] [PubMed]

29. Spiteri, T.; Newton, R.U.; Binetti, M.; Hart, N.H.; Sheppard, J.M.; Nimphius, S. Mechanical determinants of faster change of direction and agility performance in female basketball athletes. *J. Strength Cond. Res.* **2015**, *29*, 2205–2214. [CrossRef] [PubMed]

30. Spiteri, T.; Nimphius, S.; Hart, N.H.; Specos, C.; Sheppard, J.M.; Newton, R.U. Contribution of strength characteristics to change of direction and agility performance in female basketball athletes. *J. Strength Cond. Res.* **2014**, *28*, 2415–2423. [CrossRef] [PubMed]

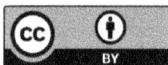

sports

MDPI

Article

Outcomes following Hip and Quadriceps Strengthening Exercises for Patellofemoral Syndrome: A Systematic Review and Meta-Analysis

Adebisi Bisi-Balogun * and Firdevs Torlak

Clinical Exercise Science, Faculty of Health Science, University of Potsdam Out-Patient Clinic, Potsdam 14469, Brandenburg, Germany; torlak@uni-potsdam.de
* Correspondence: bisibalo@uni-potsdam.de; Tel./Fax: +49-157-5721-2035

Academic Editor: Lee E. Brown
Received: 20 September 2015; Accepted: 21 October 2015; Published: 23 October 2015

Abstract: There is growing evidence to support change in the rehabilitation strategy of patellofemoral pain syndrome (PFPS) from traditional quadriceps strengthening exercises to inclusion of hip musculature strengthening in individuals with PFPS. Several studies have evaluated effects of quadriceps and hip musculature strengthening on PFPS with varying outcomes on pain and function. This systematic review and meta-analysis aims to synthesize outcomes of pain and function post-intervention and at follow-up to determine whether outcomes vary depending on the exercise strategy in both the short and long term. Electronic databases including MEDLINE, EMBASE, CINAHL, Web of Science, PubMed, Pedro database, Proquest, Science direct, and EBscoHost databases were searched for randomized control trials published between 1st of January 2005 and 31st of June 2015, comparing the outcomes of pain and function following quadriceps strengthening and hip musculature strengthening exercises in patients with PFPS. Two independent reviewers assessed each paper for inclusion and quality. Means and SDs were extracted from each included study to allow effect size calculations and comparison of results. Six randomized control trials met the inclusion criteria. Limited to moderate evidence indicates that hip abductor strengthening was associated with significantly lower pain post-intervention (SMD -0.88, -1.28 to -0.47 95% CI), and at 12 months (SMD -3.10, -3.71 to -2.50 95% CI) with large effect sizes (greater than 0.80) compared to quadriceps strengthening. Our findings suggest that incorporating hip musculature strengthening in management of PFPS tailored to individual ability will improve short-term and long-term outcomes of rehabilitation. Further research evaluating the effects of quadriceps and hip abductors strengthening focusing on reduction in anterior knee pain and improvement in function in management of PFPS is needed.

Keywords: anterior knee pain; function; hip; muscle strengthening; muscle endurance

1. Introduction

Patello-femoral pain syndrome (PFPS) is one of the most diagnosed knee pain syndromes in paediatric physical therapy or orthopaedic outpatient clinics [1–3] and is thus implicated as the primary cause of knee pain in clinical settings in up to 40% of cases [4,5]. PFPS is prevalent in active young adults with a noticeable peak of prevalence in young, active adolescents between the ages of 12 and 17 years with double the annual incidence in women compared to men [1–3].

Diagnosis and treatment of PFPS poses a challenge in clinical practice, as its exact aetiology is unknown. However, PFPS describes anterior knee pain resulting from several intrinsic factors including increased Q-angle in the weight-bearing position, genu valgus, tibia internal rotation, patellar mal-alignment, muscular imbalance around the hip and knee joints, and over-activity [6].

Thus, diagnosis of PFPS requires exclusion of other conditions including intra-articular pathologic abnormality, plica syndromes, Osgood-Schlatter disease, neuromas, and other rare causes [6,7].

Conservative management options, which have been suggested for PFPS, include quadriceps strengthening, stretching, bracing, and patella taping although no specific intervention has been reported to be most effective in management of PFPS [8–10]. Quadriceps strengthening in the management of PFPS has been the focus of clinical interventions to correct patella tracking, alignment, and motion seen in PFPS thus reducing resultant increased patellar joint pressure and pain [8,10]. However, abnormal hip motion in both frontal and transverse planes due to weak hip muscles occurs in PFPS further influencing pain, knee kinematics, and function [9]. Poor eccentric hip abductors and external rotator muscle strength causes a resultant femoral adduction and medial rotation during weight-bearing activities, causing a lateral patellar tracking as the femur medially rotates beneath the patella, resulting in patellar mal-alignment [10,11].

Studies have reported that when compared to healthy controls, persons with PFPS show deficits in hip abductor, extensor, and external rotator muscle strength [12,13]. A deficit in hip abductor strength deficit compared with healthy controls of up to 14% has been reported in persons with PFP syndrome, resulting in impaired medial–lateral postural stability with diminished quantitative balance performance difference of up to 39%–45% [14]. This strength deficit plays huge biomechanical significance as seen in diminished single leg stance performance with following fatiguing of the hip abductor muscles [15] and also a reported correlation between balance performance and hip muscle abductor strength in adults [16]. The gluteus medius is an important muscle in controlling frontal-plane motion in a far reaching movement of the arm compared to ankle evertors and invertors, and as such play a significant role in maintaining normal posture in response to medial-lateral perturbations on the body [17].

The primary goals in management of PFPS, either surgical or conservative management, are the reduction in intensity of anterior knee pain, and restoration of patient optimal function (aspects of interaction between a person's health status and their contextual factors either environmental and personal factors) [8,13]. Evaluation of pain intensity and function pre and post intervention, provides a means of determining whether goals of conservative management of PFPS are achieved and serve as a means of assessing severity of patient symptoms at different time points during the course of management [8].

Although several studies have focused on the effects of both quadriceps strengthening and hip abductor strengthening on pain, hip muscle function and functional activities in PFPS reported mixed and inconclusive results.

Therefore, this meta-analysis was aimed to:

a. Determine differences in patient-reported anterior knee pain intensity in management of PFPS following quadriceps strengthening or hip abductor strengthening programs in management of PFPS.

b. Determine differences in function following quadriceps strengthening or hip abductor strengthening programs in management of PFPS.

2. Materials and Methods

2.1. Type of Participants

Studies were included if they reported having both male and female participants aged 15 to 40 years with a diagnosis of PFPS by medical and radiographic examination.

2.2. Types of Studies

Studies selection was limited to randomized control trial studies to reflect the highest level of clinical research quality. All studies reported pre and post intervention data of outcomes of anterior knee pain intensity and function following quadriceps strengthening and hip abductor strengthening programs in management of PFPS.

2.3. Type of Interventions

The interventions under consideration were quadriceps strengthening alone or hip abductor and external rotator strengthening programme in management of PFPS.

2.4. Outcome Measurements

Outcome measures used in selected studies in this review to evaluate pain and function included:

- Function—Evaluated with outcome measures including lower extremity function score (LEFS), Western Ontario and McMaster Universities Arthritis Index (WOMAC), or anterior knee pain score (AKPS), which have all been consistently used in research to assess function of the lower extremity pre and post intervention in management of PFPS [8].
- Pain as measured with outcome measures including the visual analogue scale or numerical pain rating scale (0/10) which have both been consistently used in research to assess anterior knee pain intensity pre and post intervention, in management of PFPS [3,8].

Validity and Reliability of Outcome Measures

Reliability for the LEFS and AKPS has been reported to be $R = 0.98$ and $R = 0.95$ in subjects with PFPS [18]. Reliability and validity of outcome measures of pain selected for this study, including the visual analogue scale (VAS) and numerical pain rating scale (NPRS) have been described in literature.

The VAS and the NPRS compared to other pain rating tools has a better responsiveness compared to other rating tools with an inter-rater reliability of $ICC = 0.76$ and 0.84 respectively [3,8].

2.5. Electronic Search

An electronic online search was conducted using a systematic search strategy to identify relevant articles in electronic databases including MEDLINE, EMBASE, CINAHL, Web of Science, PubMed, Pedro database, Proquest, Science direct, and EBscoHost for studies published in English between 2008 and May 2015 to reflect current research knowledge. Key word combinations used included: patellofemoral pain syndrome, anterior knee pain, function, hip, muscle strengthening, and muscle endurance. The electronic data search was limited to randomized control trial studies only to reflect the highest level of clinical research quality included in this review. In addition, a manual searching of the references of all articles selected for the review and bibliographies of relevant texts and journals was conducted. Depositories of unpublished research were not perused and although the authors agree this may potentially lead to publication bias [19], it is impossible to exhaustively peruse all unpublished work on effects of strength training interventions associated with PFPS from all authors and institutions around the world related to this research area.

2.6. Inclusion and Exclusion Criteria

Inclusion Criteria—Studies with

- Participants aged 15–40 years.
- Comparison of pre and post intervention outcomes following quadriceps strengthening or hip abductor strengthening programs in management of PFPS including anterior knee pain and patient reported function.
- Incidence of PFPS of at-least four weeks onset. Participants had to report anterior, retro, or peri-patellar pain during at least two or three of the following provocative activities: squatting, kneeling, prolonged sitting, ascending or descending stairs, running, hopping, jumping, palpation or compression of medial or lateral patella facet, and isometric quadriceps contraction.

- Studies published between 1st of January 2005 and 31st of June 2015.

   Exclusion criteria

O   Studies were excluded if they reported inclusion of participants with a previous history of knee surgeries, lower limb pathology, or dysfunctions including knee/patellar osteoarthritis, bursitis, meniscal injuries and knee collateral or cruciate ligament injuries, or other pathological diseases of the knee joint.

2.7. Study Selection

Two reviewers independently performed the process of study selection based on the title and the abstract. Articles not excluded by both reviewers were assessed in full-text and disagreement regarding inclusion was resolved by consensus.

Quality Rating of Selected Studies

For studies meeting inclusion criteria, the PEDRO scale was used to appraise their methodological quality. It has a fair inter-rater agreement for individual domains and substantial agreement for the final grade in contrast to similar rating tools (ICC = 0.56–0.68) [19]. This was independently applied by two reviewers, with discrepancies resolved during a consensus meeting.

2.8. Data Abstraction

Data relating to study design, participants, PFPS definitions, and protocol for exercise intervention (frequency, intensity, type, and time) were extracted from all studies. The mean differences of pre and post intervention for anterior knee pain using the Visual Analogue Scale/Numerical Pain rating Scale were determined. Similarly, pre and post intervention mean differences of outcome measures of function of the lower extremity using the Anterior Knee Pain Scale (AKPS), Lower Extremity Function Scale (LEFS) and WOMAC (The Western Ontario and McMaster Universities Arthritis Index) questionnaires between subjects with PFPS in both quadriceps strengthening group and hip abductor and external rotator groups were extracted. If data were missing, information was requested from the authors to allow effect size (ES) calculations.

2.9. Data Analysis

The Cochrane review statistical program Revman 5.3 was used for statistical data analysis of effect size, heterogeneity, and Standard Error of Effect size estimate. Data were pooled for pain with the VAS and where studies evaluated lower extremity function, results were pooled using functional outcome measures for the lower extremity function variable. Calculated individual or pooled ES were categorised as small (=0.59), medium (0.60–1.19) or large (=1.20). The level of statistical heterogeneity for pooled data was established using the Chi^2 and I^2 statistics (with heterogeneity defined as $p < 0.05$). Thus, the summary measure of treatment effect was the between-groups difference in mean levels of post intervention pain reduction and increase in function, expressed as a standardised mean difference (SMD) using Hedges' (adjusted) g, which includes a correction term for sample size bias [20] Statistical heterogeneity was assessed by the I^2 test, which describes the percentage of variability among effect estimates beyond that expected by chance. Heterogeneity can be considered as unlikely to be important for I^2 values up to 40%. In the absence of statistical heterogeneity (I^2 less than or equal to 40%), individual effect sizes were combined statistically using the inverse variance random-effects method, which assumes that true effects are normally distributed [21]. Levels of evidence definitions employed in this study were as recommended by van Tulder *et al.* [22].

3. Results

The literature search produced a total of 402 studies. Six randomized control trials met the inclusion and exclusion criteria for this review. Manual search of literature sources did not produce any additional study. The search strategy is itemized in Figure 1 below.

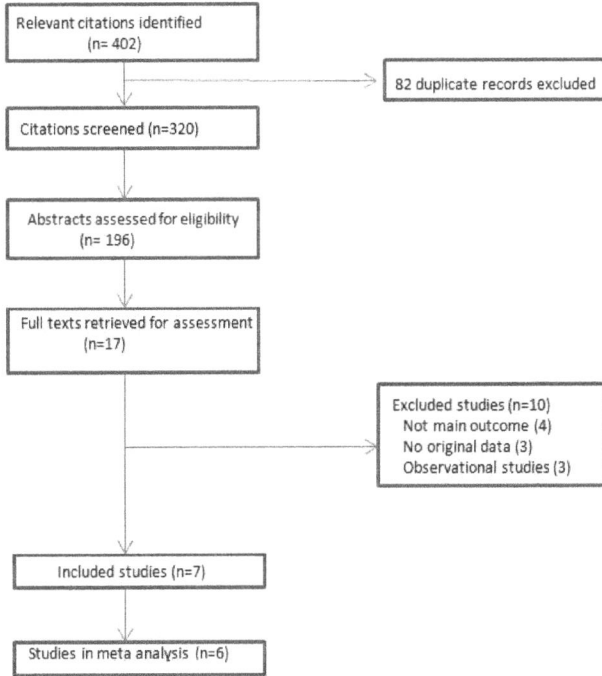

Figure 1. Flow chart showing search strategy.

3.1. Study Characteristics

A total of six randomized controlled trials met the inclusion and exclusion criteria and were included in the review. All six studies [23–28] evaluated anterior knee pain intensity (VAS/NPRS 0/10) as a pre and post intervention outcome measure. A total of four studies examined function using the functional assessment tools AKPS [25,26], LEFS [25,26,28] and WOMAC [27]. All six studies randomized a total of 214 participants (89.7% female), with sample size ranging from 14 to 54 subjects. The mean age of studies populations ranged from 16 to over 40 years. Participant eligibility was determined by clinician diagnosis of PFPS of at least four weeks onset, and a fulfilment of an inclusion and exclusion criteria as itemized in Table 1. Interventions typically involved exercising for three 30–45 min sessions per week for 4-8 weeks, a range of 12–24 sessions per trial [23–28].

Table 1. Description of Methods and characteristics of included studies with quality ratings score.

Author	Study Population/Group Allocation	Inclusion/Exclusion Criteria	Follow up/Monitoring	Intervention Description	Pre and Post-Operative Measurements	Randomisation Process	Pedro Score (0/10)
Nagakawa et al. 2008 [23] RCT	14 subjects (4 male; 10 females): QUADSG (7) HABLG (7)	Inclusion—Clinically diagnosed with PFP; anterior knee pain; insidious onset of pain unrelated to a traumatic incident and persistent for at least four weeks; presence of pain on palpation of the patellar facets. Exclusion—Intra-articular pathologic conditions; cruciate or collateral ligament involvement; tenderness over patellar tendon, iliotibial band, or pes anserinus tendon; patellar apprehension; Osgood-Schlatter or Sinding-Larsson-Johansson syndromes; hip or lumbar referred pain; a history of patellar dislocation; knee effusion; or previous patellofemoral joint surgery.	No follow-up period	Duration—5 sessions/week for 6 weeks, 1 supervised and 4 unsupervised weekly session. QUADSG— 1. Open and closed kinetic chain exercises for quadriceps strengthening, 2. Sitting hamstring stretch, 3 repetitions/30-s hold; patellar mobilization, Standing quadriceps, calf and iliotibial band stretch. 3. Isometric quadriceps contractions while sitting with 90° of knee flexion 2 sets of 10 repetitions/10-s hold 4. Straight-leg raise in supine position 3 sets of 10 repetitions 5. Mini squats to 40° of knee flexion 4 sets of 10 repetitions Balance training 3 sets. HABSG—Same as QUADSG with addition of 1. Transversus abdominis muscle contraction in the quadruped position 2 sets of 15 repetitions/10-s hold. 2. Isometric combined hip abduction-lateral rotation in side-lying and then quadruped position with the hips using elastic resistance 2 sets of 15 repetitions/10-s hold for each position. 3. Side-lying isometric hip abduction with extended knee 2 sets of 15 repetitions/10-s hold. 4. Additional elastic resistance around the affected leg in the forward lunges to encourage lateral rotation and abduction of the hip. All subjects performed the rehabilitation exercises once a week under the supervision of the principal investigator and four times a week at home, for a total of five sessions a week for six weeks.	Pain—Worst and usual pain; Pain during stair ascending and descending (VAS)	Sealed envelope, blinded assessors, single blinded	9

Table 1. *Cont.*

Author	Study Population/Group Allocation	Inclusion/Exclusion Criteria	Follow up/Monitoring	Intervention Description	Pre and Post-Operative Measurements	Randomisation Process	Pedro Score (0/10)
Razeghi et al. 2010 [24] RCT	32 females; mean age 22.62 ± 2.67 years (18–30); QUADSG (16) HABLG (16)	Inclusion—Clinically diagnosed with PFP; anterior knee pain; insidious onset of pain unrelated to a traumatic incident of at least four weeks onset; pain during patellar orthopaedic test or facet tenderness. Exclusion—Intra-articular pathologic conditions; cruciate or collateral ligament involvement; tenderness over iliotibial band, patella or pes anserinus tendon; patellar apprehension; Osgood-Schlatter or Sinding-Larsen-Johansson syndromes; hip or lumbar referred pain; a history of patellar dislocation; Pregnancy; history of being on a steroidal or nonsteroidal medication in last 6 months	No follow-up	Duration—4-week treatment program, supervised. QUADSG—Strengthening exercise in the control group focused only on the quadriceps muscle. The treatment program consisted of progressive resistive exercises for the hip muscles and terminal and 90° to 50° resistive knee extension and mini squat for the quadriceps. The Mc Queen progressive resistive technique was applied to increase exercise resistance. HABSG—Exercise intervention not properly described.	Usual pain measured with VAS	Random allocation	5
Fukuda et al. 2010 [25] RCT	70 females; mean age 25 years (20–40); QUADSG (22); HABSG (23) Control group (25)	Inclusion—History of anterior knee pain of more than 3 months onset; reported pain in 2 or more daily activities; sedentary for at least the past 6 months. Exclusion—Pregnant or had any neurological disorders; hip, knee, or ankle injuries; low back or sacroiliac joint pain; rheumatoid arthritis; used corticosteroids or anti-inflammatory drugs; a heart condition that prohibited performing the exercises; or previous surgery involving the lower extremities.	No follow up	Duration—3 sessions per week for 4 weeks, totalling 12 sessions, supervised. QUADSG— 1. Stretching and strengthening of knee musculature. Stretching (HM, PF, quadriceps, and ITB), 3 sets/30 s 2. Iliopsoas strengthening in non-weight bearing, 3 sets/10 repetitions. 3. Seated knee extension 90°–45°, 3 sets/10 repetitions. 4. Leg press 0°–45°, 3 sets/10 repetitions 5. Squatting 0°–45°, 3 sets/10 repetitions. HABSG—Same protocol as QUADSG, with the addition of exercises to strengthen the hip abductor and lateral rotator muscles. Standardized to 70% of the 1-repetition maximum. 1. Hip abduction against elastic band (standing), 3 sets/10 repetitions 2. Hip abduction with weights (side-lying), 3 sets/10 repetitions 3. Hip external rotation against elastic band (sitting), 3 sets/10 repetitions. 4. Side-stepping against elastic band, 3 reps/1 min.	Pain during stair ascending and descending (NPRS); Lower extremity function with LEFS and AKPS	Random allocation using opaque and sealed envelopes containing the names of the groups	8

Table 1. *Cont.*

Author	Study Population/Group Allocation	Inclusion/Exclusion Criteria	Follow up/Monitoring	Intervention Description	Pre and Post-Operative Measurements	Randomisation Process	Pedro Score (0/10)
Fukuda et al. 2012 [26] RCT	54 females; mean age 23 years QUADSG (26); HABSG (28)	Inclusion—History of anterior knee pain of more than 3 months onset; reported pain in 2 or more daily activities; sedentary for at least the past 6 months. Exclusion—Pregnant or had any neurological disorders; hip, knee, or ankle injuries; low back or sacroiliac joint pain; rheumatoid arthritis; used corticosteroids or anti-inflammatory drugs; a heart condition that prohibited performing the exercises; or previous surgery involving the lower extremities.	1 year	Duration—3 sessions per week for 4 weeks, totalling 12 sessions, supervised exercise sessions QUADSG— 1. Stretching and strengthening of the knee musculature. Stretching (HM, PF, quadriceps, and ITB), 3 sets/30 s sets/10 repetitions. 2. Iliopsoas strengthening in non-weight bearing, 3 sets/10 repetitions. 3. Seated knee extension 90°–45°, 3 sets/10 repetitions. 4. Leg press 0°–45°, 3 sets/10 repetitions. 5. Squatting 0°–45°, 3 sets/10 repetitions. HABSG—Same protocol as QUADSG, with the addition of exercises to strengthen the hip abductor and lateral rotator muscles. Standardized to 70% of the 1-repetition maximum. 1. Hip abduction against elastic band (standing), 3 sets/10 repetitions. 2. Hip abduction with weights (side-lying), 3 sets/10 repetitions 3. Hip external rotation against elastic band (sitting), 3 sets/10 repetitions. 4. Side-stepping against elastic band, 3 reps/1 min.	Pain during stair ascending and descending (NPRS); Lower extremity function with LEFS and AKPS	Random allocation using opaque and sealed envelopes containing the names of the groups	8
Khayambashis et al. 2014 [27] RCT	36 (18 male; 18 female); mean age 27.3 ± 7 years (19–35 years); QUADSG (18) HABSG (18)	Inclusion—Unilateral or bilateral PFP diagnosed by a physician. Exclusion—Ligamentous laxity; meniscal injury; pes anserine bursitis; iliotibial band syndrome; patella tendinitis; or a history of patella dislocation, patella fracture, knee surgery or symptoms that had been present for ≤6 months.	6 months	Duration—3 sessions/week for 8 weeks totalling 24 sessions; 3 sets, 20–25 reps/set, supervised exercise sessions. QUADSG— 1. Resisted knee extension using an elastic with subjects extending the knee from 30 of knee flexion to full knee extension. 2. Partial squat against resistance from the start position to full knee extension while squeezing a ball between both knees HABSG— 1. Hip abductor strengthening in side lying on a treatment table with elastic tubing providing resistance by abducting the hip from 0° to 30° 3 sets, 20–25 reps/set 2. Hip external rotator strengthening performed seated at the edge of a treatment table and the knee flexed to 90° with elastic tubing tied around the ankle providing resistance as subjects externally rotated the hip from 0° to 30°.	Usual pain (VAS); Lower extremity function (WOMAC).	Controlled clinical trial	5

Table 1. *Cont.*

Author	Study Population/Group Allocation	Inclusion/Exclusion Criteria	Follow up/Monitoring	Intervention Description	Pre and Post-Operative Measurements	Randomisation Process	Pedro Score (0/10)
Doldak *et al.* 2011 [28] RCT	33 females; aged 16–35 years; QUADSG (16) HABSG (17)	Inclusion—Clinically diagnosed with PFP; anterior knee pain; insidious onset of pain unrelated to a traumatic incident of at least four weeks onset; pain during patellar orthopaedic test or facet tenderness. Exclusion—Symptoms present for less than one month; self-reported other knee pathology; history of knee surgery within the last year; a self-reported history of patella dislocations or subluxations; and other concurrent significant injury affecting the lower extremity.	No follow up	Duration—8 weeks, 3 sessions per week. 1 supervised, 2 unsupervised at home (3 sets / 10 reps). 1st rehabilitation phase—4 weeks HABSG— 1. Standing; side-lying hip abduction and external rotation with 3%–5% body weight 2. Side-lying hip abduction and external rotation with 5%–7% body weight and quadruped hydrant QUADSG— 1. Short arc quads with 3%–7% body weight; Straight leg raises with 3%–7% body weight. 2. Terminal knee extensions with 3%–7% body weight. 2nd Phase—Both groups performed similar flexibility exercises (5–8 weeks) 1. Single-leg balance with front pull or standing on Airpex pad, (3 sets / 10 reps) 2. Lateral step-downs off a 10–20.3-cm step (3 sets of 10 repetitions) 3. Lunges to a 10–20.3-cm step; Single-leg calf raises alone or on Airex pad.	Usual pain (VAS), Lower extremity function with LEFS.	Participants were randomly assigned to a hip strengthening program (hip group) or a quadriceps strengthening program (quad group) for 4 weeks.	6

In three of the six studies, [23,25,26] the hip abductor strengthening group (HABSG) performed both hip abductor, external rotator, and quadriceps muscle strengthening exercises, while the quadriceps strengthening group (QUADSG) performed quadriceps muscle strengthening exercises alone. In the other three studies [24,27,28], the hip abductor strengthening group performed hip abductor and external rotator strengthening exercises alone, while subjects in the quadriceps strengthening group performed quadriceps strengthening exercises alone.

In four studies, all subjects performed stretching exercises as part of their exercise intervention sessions in both hip abductor strengthening groups and quadriceps strengthening groups [23–25,28], while stretching was not performed in the other two trials [26,27]. In two studies, all weekly exercise sessions were performed in a rehabilitation setting and supervised by the investigator [24–27] while in the other two of the studies [23,28], one out of five session weekly sessions [23] and one out of three weekly sessions [28] were supervised in the clinic by the investigator while all other sessions were performed by the subject at home unsupervised (Table 1). Only two of the six studies [26,27] reported a post-intervention follow-up period (6 and 12 months respectively).

3.2. Effect of Hip Abductor and Quadriceps Strengthening Exercise on Anterior Knee Pain

Post Intervention: The point estimate of effect size for each study indicated a greater reduction in PFPS amongst subjects in the hip abductor and external rotator muscle strengthening group compared with subjects in the quadriceps muscle strengthening groups post intervention (Figure 2). In four out of six trials [23,24,26,27] the post intervention difference in intensity of anterior knee pain was statistically significant between both groups ($p < 0.05$). One study reported non-statistically significant differences in post intervention usual pain [28] and in ascending pain post intervention [25]. In the presence of statistical heterogeneity (I^2 greater or equal to 40%), individual effect sizes could not be combined statistically using the inverse variance random-effects method, which assumes that true effects are not normally distributed. Synthesis of data showed evidence of high statistical heterogeneity ($I^2 = 78\%$, $p < 0.05$), and therefore effect size estimates from the three subgroups (usual pain, pain during ascending stairs, and descending stairs) could not be pooled (Figure 2).

However, from results of analysis of overall pain, focusing on usual pain as a subgroup of overall pain, analysis of estimates of effect sizes of usual pain intensity from four studies [23,24,27,28] indicated that there is moderate evidence showing that the hip abductor strengthening group compared to the quadriceps strengthening alone in management of PFPS resulted in more significant reduction in usual pain ($I^2 = 28\%$, $p = 0.24$) with a medium pooled ES (SMD −0.88, −1.28 to −0.47 95% CI) (Figure 2).

Six months follow up: In the presence of statistical heterogeneity ($I^2 = 67\%$), effect size estimates could not be pooled statistically. However, sub group analysis of inverse variance random effects showed an increase in effect size at six months follow-up from post-intervention levels between both groups in usual pain intensity (−0.87 to −1.43), during stair ascending (SMD −1.12 to −2.65 95% CI), and stair descending (SMD −1.09 to −2.50 95% CI) (Figure 3).

Twelve months follow up: In the absence of statistical heterogeneity ($I^2 = 0\%$, $p = 0.07$), synthesis of data at 12 months follow up from one high quality study [26] shows limited evidence for significant differences in pain reduction between both the hip abductor strengthening group and the quadriceps strengthening group at six months follow-up with no evidence of statistical heterogeneity among the pooled estimates and a large pooled effect size (SMD −3.10, −3.71 to −2.50 95% CI) (Figure 4). However, sub group analysis of inverse variance random effects showed a more significant increase in effect size estimates at 12 months follow-up between both groups in pain intensity during stair ascending (SMD −2.65 to −2.99 95% CI) and stair descending (SMD −2.50 to −3.22 95% CI) (Figure 4).

Study or Subgroup	HABSG Mean	SD	Total	QUADSG Mean	SD	Total	Weight	Std. Mean Difference IV, Random, 95% CI
Ascending stairs								
Fukuda et al 2012	-5.2	1.5	25	-1.3	1.2	24	10.1%	-2.82 [-3.63, -2.01]
Fukuda et al 2010	-2.2	2.3	21	-1.5	1.6	20	11.2%	-0.34 [-0.96, 0.27]
Nagakawa et al 2008	-3	3.2	7	-2.4	3.6	7	8.7%	-0.16 [-1.22, 0.89]
Subtotal (95% CI)			53			51	29.9%	-1.12 [-2.81, 0.57]
Heterogeneity: Tau² = 2.04; Chi² = 26.15, df = 2 (P < 0.00001); I² = 92%								
Test for overall effect: Z = 1.30 (P = 0.19)								
Descending stairs								
Fukuda et al 2012	-4.2	1.7	25	-1.4	0.9	24	10.7%	-2.01 [-2.71, -1.32]
Fukuda et al 2010	-2.6	2.3	21	-1	2.2	20	11.1%	-0.70 [-1.33, -0.06]
Nagakawa et al 2008	-4.1	2.9	7	-2.8	2.7	7	8.6%	-0.43 [-1.50, 0.63]
Subtotal (95% CI)			53			51	30.4%	-1.09 [-2.07, -0.10]
Heterogeneity: Tau² = 0.59; Chi² = 9.60, df = 2 (P = 0.008); I² = 79%								
Test for overall effect: Z = 2.17 (P = 0.03)								
Usual pain								
Khayambashis et al 2014	-5.53	1.6	18	-3.64	1.39	18	10.6%	-1.23 [-1.95, -0.51]
Razeghi et al 2010	-3.3	1.5	16	-1.51	1.5	16	10.4%	-1.16 [-1.92, -0.41]
Nagakawa et al 2008	-3.6	2.6	7	-1.5	2.8	7	8.4%	-0.73 [-1.82, 0.37]
Doldak et al 2011	-2.2	2.7	13	-1.6	2.1	13	10.3%	-0.24 [-1.01, 0.53]
Subtotal (95% CI)			54			54	39.7%	-0.87 [-1.35, -0.39]
Heterogeneity: Tau² = 0.07; Chi² = 4.17, df = 3 (P = 0.24); I² = 28%								
Test for overall effect: Z = 3.54 (P = 0.0004)								
Total (95% CI)			160			156	100.0%	-1.00 [-1.54, -0.47]
Heterogeneity: Tau² = 0.56; Chi² = 40.81, df = 9 (P < 0.00001); I² = 78%								
Test for overall effect: Z = 3.70 (P = 0.0002)								
Test for subgroup differences: Chi² = 0.21, df = 2 (P = 0.90), I² = 0%								

Decrease Favouring HABSG   Decrease Favouring QUADSG

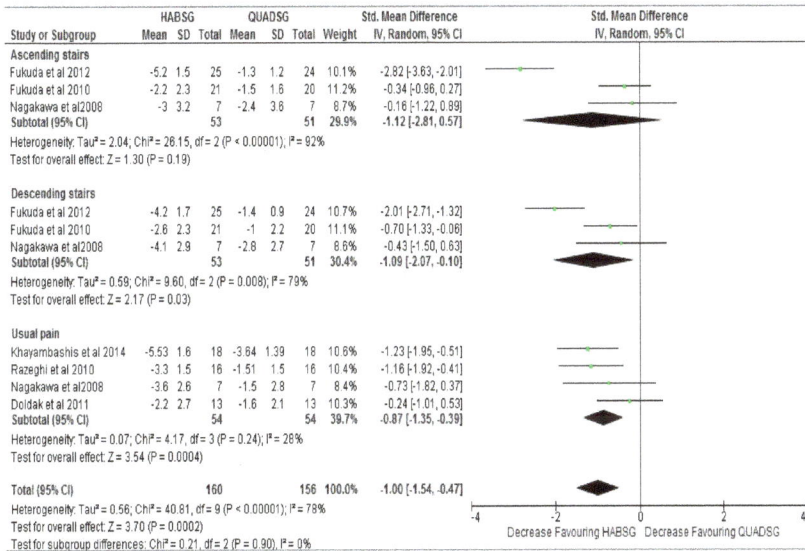

Figure 2. Post intervention: Effect size comparison and estimate of anterior knee pain intensity measured a 10 point visual analogue scale (VAS) and numerical pain rating scale (NPRS) (0/10) in both Hip abductor strengthening group (HABSG) and Quadriceps strengthening group (QUADSG).

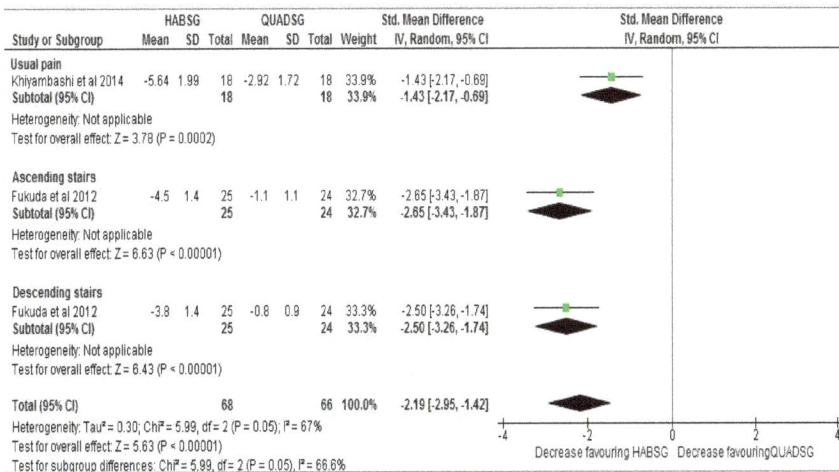

Study or Subgroup	HABSG Mean	SD	Total	QUADSG Mean	SD	Total	Weight	Std. Mean Difference IV, Random, 95% CI
Usual pain								
Khiyambashi et al 2014	-5.64	1.99	18	-2.92	1.72	18	33.9%	-1.43 [-2.17, -0.69]
Subtotal (95% CI)			18			18	33.9%	-1.43 [-2.17, -0.69]
Heterogeneity: Not applicable								
Test for overall effect: Z = 3.78 (P = 0.0002)								
Ascending stairs								
Fukuda et al 2012	-4.5	1.4	25	-1.1	1.1	24	32.7%	-2.65 [-3.43, -1.87]
Subtotal (95% CI)			25			24	32.7%	-2.65 [-3.43, -1.87]
Heterogeneity: Not applicable								
Test for overall effect: Z = 6.63 (P < 0.00001)								
Descending stairs								
Fukuda et al 2012	-3.8	1.4	25	-0.8	0.9	24	33.3%	-2.50 [-3.26, -1.74]
Subtotal (95% CI)			25			24	33.3%	-2.50 [-3.26, -1.74]
Heterogeneity: Not applicable								
Test for overall effect: Z = 6.43 (P < 0.00001)								
Total (95% CI)			68			66	100.0%	-2.19 [-2.95, -1.42]
Heterogeneity: Tau² = 0.30; Chi² = 5.99, df = 2 (P = 0.05); I² = 67%								
Test for overall effect: Z = 5.63 (P < 0.00001)								
Test for subgroup differences: Chi² = 5.99, df = 2 (P = 0.05), I² = 66.6%								

Decrease favouring HABSG   Decrease favouring QUADSG

Figure 3. At six months follow-up: Effect size comparison and estimate of anterior knee pain intensity measured with a 10 point visual analogue scale/NPRS (0/10) in both Hip abductor strengthening group (HABSG) and Quadriceps strengthening group (QUADSG).

Sports 2015, 3, 281–301

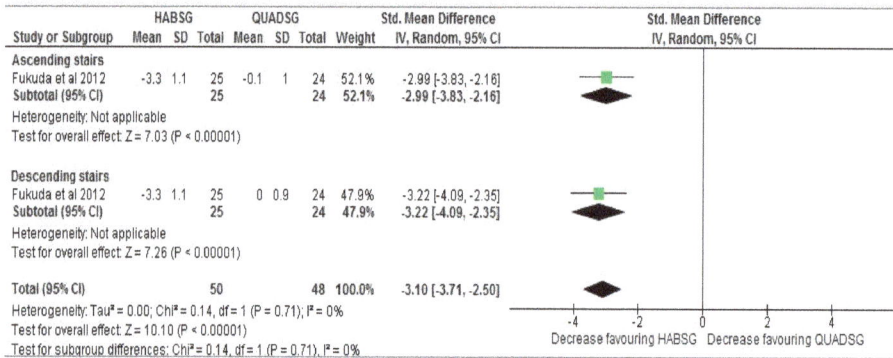

Figure 4. At 12 months follow-up: Effect size comparison and estimate of anterior knee pain intensity measured with a 10 point VAS/NPRS (0/10) in both Hip abductor strengthening group (HABSG) and Quadriceps strengthening group (QUADSG).

3.3. Effect of Hip Abductor and Quadriceps Strengthening Exercise on Function

Post intervention: Four trials evaluated function pre and post intervention. The point estimate of effect size of each study [25–27] excluding Doldak *et al.* [28] indicated a greater increase in function amongst subjects in the hip abductor strengthening group compared with subjects in the quadriceps muscle strengthening group. Contrastingly, Doldak *et al.* [28] showed a point estimate of effect size indicating a greater increase in function post-intervention in the quadriceps strengthening group compared to the hip abductor strengthening group (Figure 5). In two out of four studies [26,27] the post intervention differences in increased function between both groups were statistically significant and non-significant in the other two studies [25,28] ($p < 0.05$) (Figure 5). Synthesis of data showed evidence of high statistical heterogeneity ($I^2 = 87\%$, $p < 0.05$), and therefore effect sizes from the three subgroups (LEFS, AKPS and WOMAC) could not be pooled for further analysis.

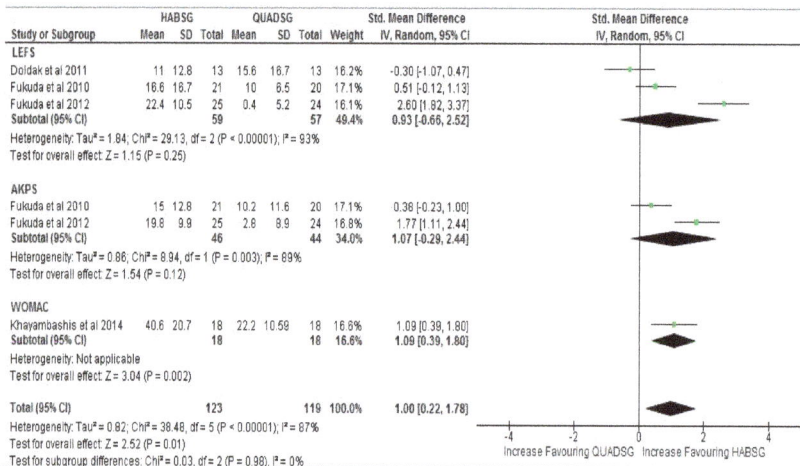

Figure 5. Post intervention: Effect size comparison of estimates of Function in subjects with Patellofemoral pain in both Hip abductor strengthening group (HABSG) and Quadriceps strengthening group (QUADSG).

Six months follow up: Due to high statistical heterogeneity ($I^2 = 66\%$, $p = 0.05$) individual effect sizes could not be combined statistically assuming that true effects are not normally distributed. Therefore, ES estimates from the three subgroups (LEFS, AKPS and WOMAC) could not be pooled (Figure 6). However, sub group analysis showed a more significant increase in effect size estimates (SMD) of function at six months follow-up from post-intervention levels between both groups in LEFS (SMD 0.99 to 2.49 95% CI); AKPS (SMD 1.07 to 1.86 95% CI); WOMAC (SMD 1.09 to 1.20 95% CI) (Figure 6).

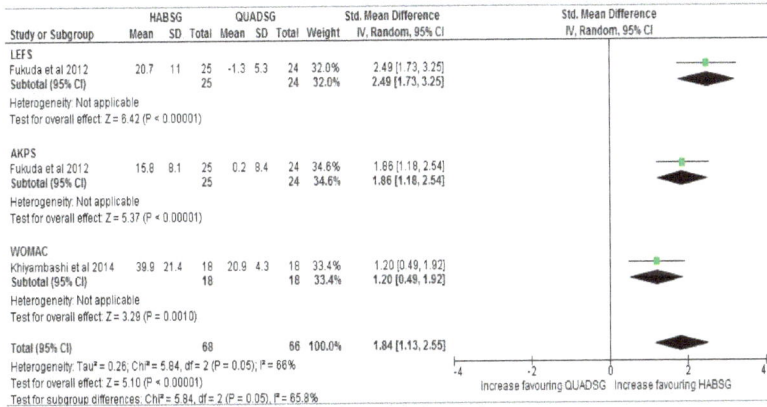

Figure 6. At six months follow-up: Effect size comparison of estimates of Function in subjects with patellofemoral pain in both Hip strengthening group (HABSG) and Quadriceps strengthening group (QUADSG).

Twelve months follow up: Due to high statistical heterogeneity ($I^2 = 65\%$, $p = 0.05$) individual effect sizes could not be combined, assuming that true effects are not normally distributed. Results from only one high quality study [26] showed a more significant increase in effect size estimates of function at from six to 12 months follow-up levels between both groups in LEFS (SMD 2.49 to 2.65 95% CI) and a slight decrease in AKPS (SMD 1.86 to 1.76 95% CI) (Figure 7).

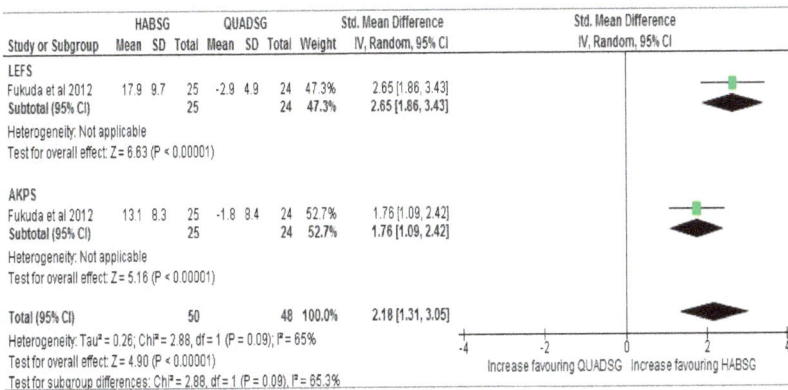

Figure 7. At 12 months follow-up: Effect size comparison and estimate of Function in subjects with patellofemoral pain in both Hip abductor strengthening group (HABSG) and Quadriceps strengthening group (QUADSG).

4. Discussion

The aim of this meta-analysis was to compare effects of hip abductor strengthening and quadriceps strengthening in management of PFPS. Results from individual studies indicated significant differences in usual pain intensity post intervention, and pain and function at six and 12 months follow-up with large effect sizes. However, these post intervention differences were not consistent in their level of statistical significances across all studies and tasks with high statistical heterogeneity of data during synthesis. While attempting to identify methodological differences to explain this disparate finding, one possible explanation could be because PFPS diagnosis is based on a group of symptoms and not a specific test. And although inclusion and exclusion criteria were similar, they differed between studies with some variability in terms of localization, onset of pain and pre-intervention level of function of subjects meeting eligibility criteria for inclusion across studies. In two studies [23,28] onset of PFPS as an inclusion criteria of participants was minimum of four weeks onset of PFPS while the four remaining studies [24–27] reported an inclusion criteria of a minimum of six months onset of PFPS (Table 1).

Due to high level of statistical heterogeneity, outcomes of overall pain post-intervention and at six months follow-up and function post intervention and at six months and 12 months follow-up were not pooled. Thus, individual effect sizes could not be combined statistically using the inverse variance random-effects method, assuming that true effects were not normally distributed across studies.

4.1. Anterior Knee Pain

Post intervention, effect sizes were medium-to-strong, indicating that the hip strengthening group demonstrated greater improvements in usual pain post intervention (Figure 2) and overall pain at 12 months follow-up (Figure 4) compared with the quadriceps strengthening group. Moderate evidence indicates that usual pain was significantly reduced in the hip abductor strengthening group compared to the quadriceps strengthening group with a moderate effect size (SMD -0.88, -1.28 to -0.47 95% CI) immediately post-intervention (analysis of a total of 108 subjects). While hip abductor strengthening exercises and quadriceps strengthening exercises reduced usual pain intensity post-intervention, there was a significant difference in the magnitude of this post-intervention usual pain reduction between both groups, with far greater pain reduction in the hip abductor strengthening groups.

At 12 months follow-up for overall pain, analysis of data (a total of 49 subjects) showed a large pooled effect size (SMD -3.10, -3.71 to -2.50 95% CI). This increased effect size estimate compared to post intervention effect sizes between both groups may be explained as a consequence of a gradual increase in overall pain post-intervention in the quadriceps strengthening group. Low evidence indicates an increased reduction in overall pain in the hip abductor strengthening group compared to the quadriceps strengthening group at 12 months follow up.

4.2. Function

Results show that the hip abductor strengthening groups showed a greater increase in function post-intervention and at six and 12 months follow-up compared to the quadriceps strengthening groups according to point estimates of effect sizes across subgroups for LEFS, AKPS [25,26,28] and WOMAC [27]. However, the magnitude of effect sizes of function between both groups became more significant at six and 12 months follow-up compared to post intervention estimates. This may be explained to be as a result of a noticeable steady decline in function in the quadriceps strengthening groups compared to the hip abductor strengthening group from post intervention levels, widening the point estimates of effect size between groups in the long term as seen from the results. Overall estimates of function could not be pooled due to heterogeneity of effect size estimates across studies. Although individual studies report increased function post intervention, no evidence exists due to statistical heterogeneity of outcomes reported.

A recently published study by Regelski *et al.* (2015) [29] reported similar outcomes post intervention and at follow-up by interpreting pooled effect sizes of individual studies post-intervention and at follow-up where applicable. However, they did not provide a clear interpretation of data as they did not perform further analysis with pooling and synthesis of data with recommendations made from effect sizes from individual studies.

4.3. Exercise Interventions

Changes in lower limb kinetics and kinematics occur in PFPS with weakness of hip muscles, a clinical finding in PFPS, associated with changes in hip and knee joint kinematics in PFPS [8–10]. Incorporating hip musculature strengthening (abductors and external rotator) into rehabilitation programs in management of PFPS may increase patient function and reduce severity of PFPS symptoms [23]. Amongst included trials, there were similarities in hip strengthening and quadriceps protocols with regards to exercise frequency: three sessions weekly for four weeks [24–26,28]. Two studies, Khayambashi *et al.* [27] and Nakagawa *et al.* [23] required patients to perform exercises three times per week for eight weeks and five times per week for six weeks, respectively. However, the types of exercises performed varied across studies. Apart from the study by Razeghi *et al.* [24] where exercise protocol was not properly described, five studies incorporated stretching of the hamstrings, quadriceps, and triceps surae as part of the PFPS protocols and used side-lying hip abduction in the hip strengthening protocol [23,25–28].

Standing hip abduction exercise was performed in three studies [25,26,28] while three studies [25–27] progressed hip abduction exercises in side-lying and standing by incorporating use of an elastic band. Four studies performed strengthening of the hip external rotation in sitting with or without the use of an elastic band [25–28]. Dolak *et al.* [28] and Nakagawa *et al.* [23] combined hip abduction and external rotation in side-lying to strengthen both abductors and external rotators. With reference to exercise types, Nakagawa *et al.* [23] used isometric exercises while the other five studies used isotonic exercises.

While there is no evidence of effects of different quadriceps strengthening and hip abductor strengthening exercise protocols influencing rehabilitation outcomes in management of PFPS, there is a possibility that this may have contributed to the high heterogeneity of pooled data across studies included in this review.

4.4. Strengths and Limitations and Recommendations

Strengths of this study include synthesis of homogenous data only where data are assumed to reflect similar effects across studies and are normally distributed. Therefore, this review not only provides data crucial to healthcare decision-making, such as uptake of hip strengthening exercise in rehabilitation strategies for PFPS, but data that are derived from trials conducted under conditions that most closely match the context of usual healthcare practice.

Limitations of this review include inclusion of a small number of studies as only the six included RCTs met the inclusion criteria. Additionally, as a result of the high heterogeneity of pooled data (I^2 greater or equal to 40%), further analysis of pooled data for overall pain post-intervention and function post-intervention and at follow-up could not be made. Future studies should systematically homogenize participant's eligibility criteria for selection of patients with PFPS to improve the quality research and consistency of outcomes in management of PFPS. While methodological quality across all studies was moderate to high with the Pedro scale, only one of the studies stated that the assessors responsible for collecting baseline and post-intervention outcomes were blinded to group assignment. Heterogeneity of reported outcomes in research on PFPS is too large to allow a clinically and scientifically sound meta-analysis of data. Better designed studies should be conducted considering limitations of currently existing studies.

In addition, valid and reliable scales, responsive to PFPS specifically, like the anterior knee pain scale (AKPS) (also known as the Kujula scale) was used by only two of the included studies [25,26]. The systematic use of the AKPS in studies on PFPS could allow optimal comparability between participants.

Sports **2015**, *3*, 281–301

PFPS is a multifactorial and complex condition and it is evident that the target population is often heterogeneous and thus could be separated in subgroups. Also, similarities and variances in exercise protocols provide a strong basis to incorporate a standardised exercise protocol and regimen for hip abductor or quadriceps strengthening exercises in conservative management of PFPS to aid future research into this condition.

5. Conclusions

Although results indicate that quadriceps strengthening may also reduce intensity of usual pain post-intervention, for greater significant post-intervention and clinically beneficial long-term outcomes, hip strengthening should be the preferred treatment approach for management of PFPS. However, there is currently low to moderate quality evidence to support this recommendation. Future studies should seek development of eligibility criteria/PFPS subject checklists for inclusion of subjects into studies on PFPS, and also take into consideration limitations of current studies so as to minimize, to the barest minimum, heterogeneity of outcomes from studies on PFPS.

Acknowledgments: The authors wish to acknowledge the authors of studies included in this review and authors who provided requested original data. We also acknowledge the staff at the Outpatient clinic, University of Potsdam.

Author Contributions: Adebisi Bisi-Balogun was tasked with preparation and finalisation of manuscript; statistical data analysis and interpretation of the results. Both authors conducted the electronic search process; quality ratings of the methodological process of included studies; data abstraction and revision of manuscript.

Conflicts of Interest: The author declares no conflicts of interest.

References

1.   Boling, M.; Padua, D.; Marshall, S.; Guskiewicz, K.; Pyne, S.; Beutler, A. Gender differences in the incidence and prevalence of patellofemoral pain syndrome. *Scand. J. Med. Sci. Sports* **2010**, *20*, c723–c730. [CrossRef] [PubMed]
2.   Blond, L.; Hansen, L. Patellofemoral pain syndrome in athletes: A 5.7-year retrospective follow-up study of 250 athletes. *Acta Orthop. Belg.* **1998**, *644*, 393–400.
3.   Callaghan, M.J.; Selfe, J. Has the incidence or prevalence of patellofemoral pain in the general population in the United Kingdom been properly evaluated? *Phys. Ther. Sport* **2007**, *81*, 37–43. [CrossRef]
4.   Wood, L.; Muller, S.; Peat, G. The epidemiology of patellofemoral disorders in adulthood: A review of routine general practice morbidity. *Prim. Health Care Res. Dev.* **2011**, *122*, 157–164. [CrossRef] [PubMed]
5.   Witvrouw, E.; Callaghan, M.J.; Stefanik, J.J.; Noehren, B.; Bazett-Jones, D.M.; Willson, J.D.; Earl-Boehm, J.E.; Davis, I.S.; Powers, C.M.; McConnell, J.; *et al.* Patellofemoral pain: Consensus statement from the 3rd International Patellofemoral Pain Research Retreat held in Vancouver, 2013. *Br. J. Sports Med.* **2014**, *48*, 411–414. [CrossRef] [PubMed]
6.   Thomee, R.; Augustsson, J.; Karlsson, J. Patellofemoral pain syndrome: A review of current issues. *Sports Med.* **1999**, *284*, 245–262. [CrossRef]
7.   Lankhorst, N.E.; Bierma-Zeinstra, S.; van Middelkoop, M. Factors associated with patellofemoral pain syndrome: A systematic review. *Br. J. Sports Med.* **2013**, *47*, 193–206. [CrossRef] [PubMed]
8.   Rothermich, M.; Glaviano, N.; Li, J.; Hart, J. Patellofemoral Pain Epidemiology, Pathophysiology, and Treatment Options. *Clin. Sports Med.* **2015**, *34*, 313–327. [CrossRef] [PubMed]
9.   Mascal, C.L.; Landel, R.; Powers, C. Management of patellofemoral pain targeting hip, pelvis, and trunk muscle function: 2 case reports. *J. Orthop. Sports Phys. Ther.* **2003**, *33*, 647–660. [CrossRef] [PubMed]
10. Powers, C.M.; Ward, S.R.; Fredericson, M.; Guillet, M.; Shellock, F.G. Patellofemoral kinematics during weight-bearing and non-weight-bearing knee extension in persons with lateral subluxation of the patella: A preliminary study. *J. Orthop. Sports Phys. Ther.* **2003**, *33*, 677–685. [CrossRef] [PubMed]
11. Ferber, R.; Davis, I.M.; Williams, D.S., III. Gender differences in lower extremity mechanics during running. *Clin. Biomech.* **2003**, *18*, 350–357. [CrossRef]

12. Bolgla, L.A.; Malone, T.R.; Umberger, B.R.; Uhl, T.L. Hip strength and hip and knee kinematics during stair descent in females with and without patellofemoral pain syndrome. *J. Orthop. Sports Phys. Ther.* **2008**, *381*, 12–18. [CrossRef] [PubMed]

13. Cichanowski, H.R.; Schmitt, J.S.; Johnson, R.J.; Niemuth, P.E. Hip strength in collegiate female athletes with patellofemoral pain. *Med. Sci. Sports Exerc.* **2007**, *398*, 1227–1232. [CrossRef] [PubMed]

14. Lee, S.; Souza, R.; Powers, C. The influence of hip abductor muscle performance on dynamic postural stability in females with patellofemoral pain. *Gait Posture* **2012**, *36*, 425–429. [CrossRef] [PubMed]

15. Gribble, P.A.; Hertel, J. Effect of hip and ankle muscle fatigue on unipedal postural control. *J. Electromyogr. Kinesiol.* **2004**, *146*, 641–646. [CrossRef] [PubMed]

16. Chang, S.H.; Mercer, V.S.; Giuliani, C.A.; Sloane, P.D. Relationship between hip abductor rate of force development and mediolateral stability in older adults. *Arch. Phys. Med. Rehabil.* **2005**, *869*, 1843–1850. [CrossRef] [PubMed]

17. Winter, D.A.; Prince, F.; Frank, J.S.; Powell, C.; Zabjek, K.F. Unified theory regarding A/P and M/L balance in quiet stance. *J. Neurophysiol.* **1996**, *756*, 2334–2343.

18. Watson, C.J.; Propps, M.; Ratner, J.; Zeigler, D.L.; Horton, P.; Smith, S.S. Reliability and responsiveness of the lower extremity functional scale and the anterior knee pain scale in patients with anterior knee pain. *J. Orthop. Sports Phys. Ther.* **2005**, *35*, 136–146. [CrossRef] [PubMed]

19. Maher, C.; Sherrington, C.; Herbert, R.D.; Moseley, A.M.; Elkins, M. Reliability of the PEDro Scale for Rating Quality of Randomized Controlled Trials. *Phys. Ther.* **2003**, *838*, 713–721.

20. Higgins, J.P.T.; Green, S. *Cochrane Handbook for Systematic Reviews of Interventions (V5.0.2)*; The Cochrane Collaboration: London, UK, 2009.

21. Hedges, L.V.; Vevea, J.L. Fixed and random effects models in meta-analysis. *Psychol. Methods* **1998**, *3*, 486–504. [CrossRef]

22. Van Tulder, M.; Furlan, A.; Bombardier, C.; Bouter, L.; Editorial Board of the Cochrane Collaboration Back Review Group. Updated method guidelines for systematic reviews in the Cochrane collaboration back review group. *Spine* **2003**, *28*, 1290–1299. [CrossRef] [PubMed]

23. Nakagawa, T.; Batista Muniz, T.; Marche, R.; Menezes Reiff, R.; Serra, F. The effect of additional strengthening of hip abductor and lateral rotator muscles in patellofemoral pain syndrome: A randomized controlled pilot study. *Clin. Rehabil.* **2008**, *22*, 1051–1060. [CrossRef] [PubMed]

24. Razeghi, M.; Etemadi, Y.; Taghizadeh, Sh.; Ghaem, H. Could Hip and Knee Muscle Strengthening Alter the Pain Intensity in Patellofemoral Pain Syndrome? *Iran. Red Crescent Med. J. IRCMJ* **2010**, *122*, 104–110.

25. Fukuda, T.; Rossetto, F.; Magalhães, E.; Fernandes Bryk, F.; Lucareli, P.R.; Carvalho, N. Short-Term Effects of Hip Abductors and Lateral Rotators Strengthening in Females with Patellofemoral Pain Syndrome: A Randomized Controlled Clinical Trial. *J. Orthop. Sports Phys. Ther.* **2010**, *40*, 736–740. [CrossRef] [PubMed]

26. Fukuda, T.; Pagotti Melo, W.; Zaffalon, B.; Rossetto, F.; Magalhães, E.; Fernandes Bryk, F.; Martin, R. Hip Posterolateral Musculature Strengthening in Sedentary Women with Patellofemoral Pain Syndrome: A Randomized Controlled Clinical Trial with 1-Year Follow-up. *J. Orthop. Sports Phys. Ther.* **2012**, *42*, 823–830. [CrossRef] [PubMed]

27. Khayambashi, K.; Fallah, A.; Movahed, A.; Bagwell, J.; Power, C. Posterolateral Hip Muscle Strengthening Versus Quadriceps Strengthening for Patellofemoral Pain: A Comparative Control Trial. *Arch. Phys. Med. Rehabil.* **2014**, *95*, 900–907. [CrossRef] [PubMed]

28. Dolak, D.; Silkman, C.; Mckeon, M.J.; Hosey, R.; Lattermann, C.; Uhl, T. Hip Strengthening Prior to Functional Exercises Reduces Pain Sooner than Quadriceps Strengthening in Females with Patellofemoral Pain Syndrome: A Randomized Clinical Trial. *J. Orthop. Sports Phys. Ther.* **2011**, *418*, 23–32. [CrossRef] [PubMed]

29. Regelski, C.; Ford, B.; Hoch, M. Hip Strengthening Compared with Quadriceps Strengthening in Conservative Treatment of Patients with Patellofemoral Pain: A Critically Appraised Topic. *Int. J. Athl. Ther. Train.* **2015**, *20*, 4–12. [CrossRef]

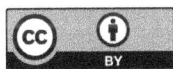

MDPI AG

St. Alban-Anlage 66

4052 Basel, Switzerland

Tel. +41 61 683 77 34

Fax +41 61 302 89 18

http://www.mdpi.com

Sports Editorial Office

E-mail: sports@mdpi.com

http://www.mdpi.com/journal/sports

www.ingramcontent.com/pod-product-compliance
Lightning Source LLC
Chambersburg PA
CBHW051316020426
42333CB00028B/3369